The 12
Dynamic Elements
of
Good Health

———

Tissue Salts

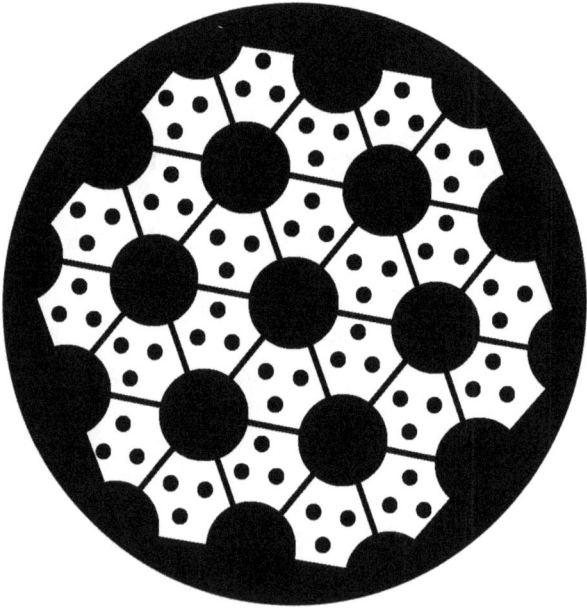

The 12 Dynamic Elements of Good Health

———

Tissue Salts

Mark Wells
Melbourne

Mark Wells
P. O. Box 79
Kew East, Vic. 3102
Australia
www.wellsnaturopathy.com.au

© Mark Wells January 1994
© Mark Wells October 1999
© Mark Wells October 2016

Editing Clean Text
Cover Design Ian Hayward
Interior Layout Cheryl Pisterman
in Minion Pro
Printed in Australia
By Mark Wells
ISBN 0 646 25990 3

Disclaimer
The information and advice contained in this book is not intended to replace the services of a qualified health professional. Consult your health professional for advice. Use of the information contained herein is beyond the control of authors and publisher, who are not responsible for any problems arising from its application.

SPECIAL THANK YOU TO:

My children, Samantha and Dean;

Angela and Ian for their support;

Bibby and Dimmy.

All my clients over the years for what they have taught me.

And of course Dr Schuessler for his original and groundbreaking
work, which introduced the Tissue Salts to the world.

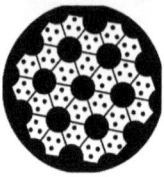

Contents

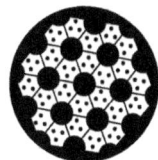

Foreword

What a privilege it is to pen the foreword for this book written by Mark Wells, my first lecturer on Dr Schuessler's Tissue Salts. My great respect for them was inspired many years ago by Mark's ability to clearly communicate how to use them in a way that realises their full healing potential. Tissue salts are a crucial intracellular food for cells and thus can nourish our whole being at the most basic level. The state of our cells expresses itself through the symptoms we experience and they indicate to us the tissue salt(s) required to recover good cell health and so overall optimal health. Mark's book is a must-read for anyone who wants to understand tissue salts well enough to enable themselves to maintain good health throughout life.

I feel honoured to be in a role that gives me the opportunity to share my understanding of tissue salts nationally and internationally. As an ambassador for the tissue salts for a large company that sells and distributes them throughout the world, I teach and educate many thousands of people about their health-promoting qualities. Mark's book always goes with me and it is the first book I recommend about tissue salts wherever my travels may take me. The book not only provides the knowledge you need to utilise tissue salts to their optimum but also makes interesting correlations with body type, diet and even astrological signs. It is never boring!

I call this book my tissue salt 'bible' and it provides all the information you need about Dr Schuessler's Tissue Salts. I share Mark's passion for tissue salts and recognise, as he does, that they are more important than ever today. Our busy lifestyle with its stresses and time constraints, and poor soils and low quality produce, all impact negatively on the quantity and quality of nutrients that reach the cells of our bodies and are absorbed by them. You can counter this negative trend by introducing tissue salts into your dietary regime. They build your body's natural immunity from the foundations – the cells – upwards.

If you want to access the immense benefits that tissue salts can provide to your ongoing health and well-being, I thoroughly recommend to you Mark's book – my 'bible' of the tissue salts.

Susan Gianevsky,
Dip T, B Ed, Dip Hom, ITF '86

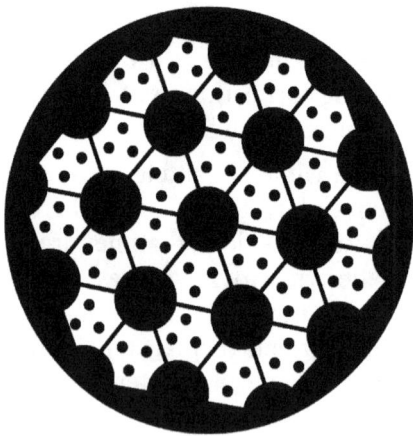

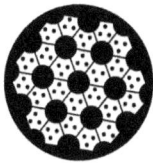

Introduction to the tissue salts

W.H. Schuessler, a German medical doctor who practised Homeopathy in the late 1800s, used basic biochemical principles to develop a practical healing science. Biochemical analysis shows that the body is composed of billions of tiny cells made up of water, organic compounds (that is, carbon-based compounds) and inorganic (non-carbon-based) minerals. Even though the bulk of the physical body is made up of water and organic compounds, minute quantities of inorganic minerals are essential activators in the continual process of repair and replacment that occurs throughout the body as cells become diseased or die. These active minerals are carried to all parts of the body in the blood, and if they are lacking or if cells have difficulty accessing, absorbing or utilising them, cell metabolism and rebuilding processes become disturbed and disease occurs.

Dr Schuessler determined that these inorganic substances are present in the body as compounds called mineral salts and he called the 12 principal compounds 'Tissue Salts'. Dr Schuessler described the types of diseases, and symptoms, arising from an imbalance or deficiency in each tissue salt, and using this knowledge, was able to prescribe with great accuracy and effect.

In order to be useful and effective, each tissue salt must be able to be absorbed quickly and efficiently into the fluid of the bloodstream and distributed to individual cells throughout the body. However, this process is not entirely straightforward, as many mineral compounds are not readily water-soluble. To facilitate absorption, Dr Schuessler prepared his tissue salt remedies using the process of *trituration*, devised by homeopaths as a way of rendering insoluble substances soluble. Trituration aims at dispersing a small amount of solids throughout a powdered medium, the way dilution disperses substances throughout a liquid medium. It involves hand-grinding 1 part mineral salt in 10 parts powdered lactose over six successive 'attenuations'. The end result is a microscopic amount of potentised tissue salt which is very readily absorbed into the bloodstream and cells of the body with NO toxic side effects.

When absorption and assimilation of tissue salts is facilitated in this way, the body is also 're-educated' in how to take up minerals from food sources more efficiently. For instance, many people, especially women, have low blood iron levels because they are unable assimilate iron properly, despite the fact that their diet contains food with a substantial iron content. In this situation, Ferrum Phosphate tissue salt confers a double benefit by providing easily absorbed iron and improving absorption of iron from food sources.

The 5 Principles of Biochemistry (as proposed by Dr Schuessler):

- Disease does not occur if cell metabolism is normal.
- Cell metabolism is normal if cell nutrition is adequate.
- Nutritional substances in the body are either of an organic or inorganic nature.
- The ability of the body's cells to assimilate and utilise nutrients, and excrete wastes, is impaired if there is an imbalance or deficiency in the inorganic mineral (tissue salt) constituent of cellular tissues.
- Adequate cell nutrition may be restored and cellular metabolism normalised by supplying the required tissue salts to the organism in a finely divided and easily assimilated form.

Tissue salts restore the balance of inorganic minerals in cell tissues, thus alleviating the symptoms of disease and in most cases removing its cause. However, if the cause of disturbance of the metabolism is not eliminated, the disease and its symptoms may return. For example, if illness has an emotional basis – as when stress plays a big part – tissue salts may restore chemical balance and improve overall resilience, but cannot address the emotional problems or life circumstances which are the root cause of the disease. Use of *Flower Essences* may be appropriate in such cases.

The three main differences between tissue salts and pharmaceutical drugs are:

1. Tissue salts are safe and without side-effects – ***non-toxic.***
2. They assist the body to heal itself by enhancing and supporting the natural innate healing potential within us all – ***non-habit forming.***
3. They encourage the body to function at its optimum (not just be symptom free) – ***improve health and well-being.***

What are tissue salts?

Tissue salts are inorganic mineral substances, exactly the same as those which compose our earth and its soils. Dr Schuessler regarded them as the material basis of the organs and tissues of the body. He came to this conclusion when he found that after combustion, these salts form the ashes of human tissue. He believed that their presence in correct balance in living tissue is a prerequisite for good health. The twelve tissue salts have been among remedies used by homeopaths since early in the 19th century, but it was Dr Scheussler who in the 1870s elevated them to the status of a complete system of healing.

How do tissue salts differ from other minerals?

In their crude state, for example as they occur in some foods, minerals are found as tightly-packed concentrates, not easily assimilated 'as is' by cell tissues: they must by broken down in the gut. However, digestive systems of individuals differ in their capacity to do this, and so absorption of mineral salts is variable. The process of hand grinding or trituration frees and disperses minerals – a sort of molecular redistribution – within a neutral medium. Trituration and attenuation appear to make minerals more acceptable to individual cells by approaching more closely the minute concentrations in which they already exist within the cell. In other words, in tissue salt form, minerals require no more breaking down and are in effect 'predigested'. In cases of deficiency or improper metabolism of particular minerals, administration of tissue salts will significantly increase uptake by cells and improve efficiency of utilisation.

What can they do?

According to Dr Schuessler, any disturbance in uptake or metabolism of the twelve essential mineral sales can lead to deficiency or relative imbalance within cells. This leads to disease conditions such as coughs, colds, asthma, gastrointestinal disturbances, circulatory disorders, slow healing and tendency to infection, skin disorders, hair and nail deterioration, hormonal imbalance, headache, insomnia, nerve-related problems, fatigue, etc. All these disease conditions have been successfully treated by administration of appropriate tissue salts, rectifying deficiency and re-establishing proper mineral balance in body tissues.

How are they administered?
How often and when?

Tissue salts are administered as a homeopathically prepared micro dose, most commonly in the form of a lactose-calcium based pill, or in liquid form in an alcohol and distilled water base.

Tissue salts are most commonly taken 4 times daily, before meals and at bedtime. However, frequency of dose may vary according to individual circumstances. Please refer to acute and chronic prescription guidelines below.

It is best not to take tissue salts immediately before or after food. If there is food or any other strong flavour in the mouth at the same time as taking remedies orally it can to some degree inhibit efficient uptake. For best results chew the tissue salt tablet and let it remain in the mouth for around 30-60 seconds before swallowing.

Are tissue salts safe?
Do they produce any side effects?

Physiologically, tissue salts are completely safe. Toxicity is not possible at such microscopic concentrations, i.e. one part per million.

There are NO side effects like those experienced when taking some pharmaceutical drugs. However, on rare occasions an individual may experience oversensitivity or idiosyncratic reaction to a tissue salt in the same way as is possible with food or any harmless substance that is ingested.

In acute illnesses there can sometimes be a brief and short-lived increase in intensity of symptoms after administering tissue salts. This is a sign that the disease process is moving rapidly to completion, and discomfort of the condition will soon be resolved. For example, in fever and inflammatory conditions it occasionally happens that after taking appropriate tissue salts, symptoms may briefly intensify, say for half an hour in the case of a child's fever,* and then rapidly improve as the disease quickly approaches resolution. Disease processes are allowed to run a natural course, the body successfully negotiates its attempts at reaching a more harmonious balance and better general health is ensured. Because of the minute doses involved, minerals can never become toxic in tissue salt form. Anyone can safely prescribe for minor ailments, gaining experience and knowledge towards more and more effective therapy. Of course, for serious illnesses, please do not hesitate to contact your qualified health practitioner. (See note on consultation of qualified practitioners regarding symptoms marked with an * under the heading 'How to use this book'.)

How long is it necessary to keep taking them?

The length of time one needs to take tissue salts is directly related to the length of time a health problem has existed. A very conservative estimate has been made allowing one month's treatment with tissues salts for every year the problem has been in existence. This estimate may seem even more conservative given the fact that more than one tissue salt is used in most treatments, combined with other supportive measures and health modalities. Nevertheless it is a reminder that true cure comes through a process. Not a miracle! See also below, prescribing for acute and chronic conditions.

How many can be taken at one time?

In general between 3 and 5 tissue salts are prescribed in an individual treatment for long-standing problems. For acute problems of recent origin fewer are prescribed as the symptoms are usually much more well-defined. One or two remedies will often be clearly indicated. The bottom line is this: tissue salts are prescribed to bring certain minerals back into proper balance in the body. It is not a matter of covering all possible options by prescribing all twelve salts. A prescriber's skill lies in recognising which minerals are out of balance in the body based on presenting symptoms, the only reliable guide. Best results are achieved by following this rationale.

How do I prescribe for acute illness?

In acute conditions where disease has developed suddenly – sudden fevers,* sudden gut or muscle pain,* physical trauma,* or for short-term conditions – head cold and 'flu etc. lasting a few hours or a few days, tissue salts are administered frequently. Remedies are taken at least 4 times daily and very often every 2 hours. They can be safely taken at 10 minute intervals in acute conditions. There is usually no need to continue once an acute episode is over.

How do I prescribe for chronic (long-term) illness?

In chronic or long-term health problems* such as recurring infections, periodic headaches or migraines, rheumatic and arthritic problems, or long-term respiratory, circulatory and skin conditions, tissue salts are usually taken 4 times daily for a number of months, the period of treatment depending on the length of time the problem has existed, and on the depth of the problem.

In long-term tissue salt treatment there may be occasional 'acute' episodes of illness.* In this case it is sometimes best to stop for a time and either administer appropriate tissue salts for the current acute episode until symptoms subside, or if discomfort is not too severe, simply wait and allow it to run its brief course. Then resume long-term treatment. Remember that tissue salts are always working with and supporting the body to achieve a better state of health. When acute episodes occur, it is the body's healing wisdom allowing an exacerbation of symptoms as a necessary stage on the path to a better quality of health. For example, someone who has suffered chronic sinus congestion may, in the initial stages of treatment with tissue salts, experience a few days of fluent nasal discharge. This can be understood as drainage of a chronically congested area of the body, and in most cases the person actually feels better despite temporary inconvenience.

It should be noted that the same tissue salt can be indicated in both acute and long-term conditions. Symptoms will be a guide.

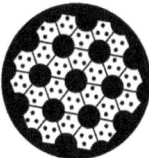

How to use this book

The purpose of this book is to give people an opportunity to experience the health-enhancing qualities of the twelve tissue salts. It is intended as a practical guide to prescribing, enabling readers to choose the most appropriate tissue salts for themselves and others, and so become empowered to take more responsibility for personal health and well-being.

Although tissue salts themselves are completely safe, many physical and mental symptoms described here may have serious consequences if not treated correctly. For this reason the book should not be seen as a replacement for seeking the advice of a qualified health professional. An asterisk* has been placed alongside descriptions of serious or potentially serious health conditions. A qualified health professional must be consulted if there is any doubt about the nature or cause of symptoms. The author has taken every care to provide accurate information for proper use of tissue salts, but cannot take any responsibility for health problems of those using this book.

About the tissue salts

This section is intended both as an introduction for the novice and a clarification for more experienced users of tissue salts. Questions about remedies are answered by the author out of many years of experience as a practitioner and teacher, and in consultation with colleagues and the work of fellow writers in the field including, naturally, Dr Schuessler.

Guide to symptomatic prescribing

At the back of the book you will find a section that lists symptoms and tissue salts appropriate to them. Remember that remedies will be most effective when prescribed on the basis of the widest possible symptom picture.

Names

Tissue salts are usually called by the abbreviations of their Latin names. At the head of each chapter this abbreviation is given, and below it the chemical name of the mineral to which it refers. These two naming systems will be used throughout the text to distinguish between a potentised tissue salt (Latin abbreviation) and its raw mineral form (chemical name). For interest, each salt's full Latin name and the mineral's common name are included in the following list:

Calc Fluor: calcium fluoride
(Calcarea Fluorica; fluoride of lime)

Calc Phos: calcium phosphate
(Calcarea Phosphorica; phosphate of lime)

Calc Sulp: calcium sulphate
(Calcarea Sulphurica; gypsum)

Ferrum Phos: iron phosphate
(Ferrum Phosphoricum; iron phosphate)

Kali Mur: potassium chloride
(Kali Muriaticum; chloride of potash)

Kali Phos: potassium phosphate
(Kali Phosphoricum; phosphate of potash)

Mag Phos: magnesium phosphate
(Magnesia Phosphorica; phosphate of magnesia)

Nat Mur: sodium chloride
(Natrum Muriaticum; common salt)

Nat Phos: sodium phosphate
(Natrum Phosphoricum; phosphate of soda)

Nat Sulph: sodium sulphate
(Natrum Sulphuricum; Glauber's salt)

Silica: silicon dioxide
(Silicea; quartz)

Arrangement of information

The first paragraph of each chapter locates places in the body where the mineral from which the tissue salt under discussion is most concentrated and gives a general description of the effects of long-term deficiency or imbalance. Subsequent subheadings are as follows:

Body type

Gives common symptom pictures and physical traits of those who respond favourably to the tissue salt under discussion. These people are particularly sensitive because of an innate tendency to deficiency or imbalance, but it should be remembered that one does not necessarily have to fit this 'classical' picture to benefit from taking the tissue salt.

Mind, head, etc.

Information under these subheadings relates to common mental characteristics and physical symptoms that develop in specific areas under conditions of imbalance and deficiency requiring tissue salts.

General
Worse by / Better by

These subheadings describe internal and external circumstances that have an ameliorating or aggravating effect on general well-being and specific symptoms of people who could benefit from the tissue salt under discussion. Anything that affects metabolism of the mineral from which the tissue salt is made will bring about these effects.

Complementary and related salts

Complementary tissue salts act synergistically – their individual properties are enhanced when they are used together. They may cover different aspects of the same function the way Silica and Calc Phos do in balancing the formation of body structure, or closely related qualities may reinforce each other, as do those of Calc Phos and Mag Phos to provide basic materials of bone structure. A synergetic effect may be created by differences in action or by overlapping actions of tissue salts.

Related tissue salts are very close in action and function. They may be considered as appropriate alternatives to each other, or as reinforcements of each other's action. For example, both Mag Phos and Calc Phos have an anti-spasmodic effect. The two may be differentiated on the basis of a wider symptom-picture where this is available, but they may also be administered together to reinforce the desired anti-spasmodic action.

Supportive measures

This section explores ways of enhancing and supporting the healing action of tissue salts. Appropriate activities, therapeutic techniques, adaptions to lifestyle and the development of new life skills can help maximise your response to tissue salts and maintain the better health that is achieved. Information presented under subsequent headings 'Diet' and 'Flower Essences' can be viewed as belonging to these supportive measures.

Diet

This section lists foods, including herbs, that not only contain significant amounts of the mineral from which a tissue salt is made, but also provide it in a relatively accessible form. Many foods contain large amounts of a particular mineral, for example dairy products with their high calcium content, but equally important is a mineral's availability for assimilation, and long experience in naturopathic practice brings into doubt the popular belief that dairy products are the best source of calcium.

Herbs must be prescribed by a qualified herbal practitioner. Correct dosage is essential, and some herbs are contra-indicated under certain circumstances.

Flower essences

Flower essences listed are those that the author has found in practice to be particularly appropriate for use in conjunction with tissue salts. They may complement the action of tissue salts by encouraging changes to mental and emotional patterns that are sources of imbalance on the physical level. It is impossible to initiate healing without reference to these subtle levels of being, and while flower essences are by no means the only way to influence mental and emotional states, they are a way that is certainly safe and gentle. Abbreviations after the names of individual essences refer to flower essence groups as follows: 'Bach': Bach Flower Remedies; 'FES': Flower Essence Society; 'Aus Bush': Australian Bush Flower Essences.

Related disciplines

Information under the headings 'Iridology' and 'Astrology' is intended to make it possible to relate information available in those fields to the use of tissue salts.

Iridology

This section relates tissue salts to particular manifestations in the iris. Iris markings are described primarily according to the author's experience in private practice, informed by the art and science of iridology – iris diagnosis. A basic knowledge of iridology is required in order to make full use of this information. If you haven't encountered this discipline before and have any doubts or are just plain fascinated, consult a qualified practitioner.

Astrology

Any tool that can provide some guidance to appropriate prescription of tissue salts is worth considering. It is not usually useful to prescribe a tissue salt on the basis of astrological correlation alone, but an individual's astrological sun sign can be included alongside iris diagnosis, tongue presentation and nail growth patterns in order to cross-reference these indicators, whose usefulness on their own is limited. In practice, the author finds that 80-85% of patients find the tissue salt associated with their sun sign useful. Though anecdotal, these figures seem to be confirmed by the experience of other practitioners. It should be noted that there are many aspects besides the sun sign that contribute to the total astrological makeup of a person.

Keywords

Keywords indicate core issues common to all subheadings. They express key characteristics addressed by a particular tissue salt. Imbalances in these areas are the primary colours from which many different shades of symptom detail are mixed!

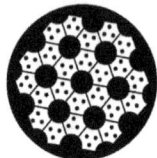

Calc Fluor

Calcium fluoride

Calcium fluoride is found in bone surfaces and tooth enamel and is also an important constituent of the elastic fibres of skin, muscular and connective tissue and the walls of blood vessels. Problems in these areas, especially related to loss of elasticity, are indicative of a metabolic disturbance involving this material.

Body type

There is a tendency towards hyper-mobility or laxness of the joints. This may manifest as great suppleness, or as proneness to sprains and strains, especially in elbows and hands, knees and ankles.

Those with a long-standing need for Calc Fluor may have teeth that are small, irregularly arranged and with enamel of poor quality. Asymmetry, particularly in the shape of the head, is not uncommon.

Mind

The hyper-mobile body can be a reflection of a 'hyper'-mobile mind. In the positive state, a person can be very creative, imaginative and not limited by rigid constraints of conventional thought. In the negative state, the picture might be that of the unstable child at school with a mind that constantly wanders, or a person who constructs exaggerated fantasies about life to avoid the confinement of reality. A mind lacking boundaries and tone may burn out, forget easily and become depressed. As with all calcium imbalances, anxieties may arise.

Head and face

Growths and swellings (e.g. cysts under the skin) of stony hardness may indicate a need for Calc Fluor.

Eyes

Blurred vision,*or just a delay in focus when looking around, suggests a lack of tone in the visual apparatus and may indicate a need for Calc Fluor. Also for cataract,*or for hard cysts in the area of the eyes, think of Calc Fluor combined with Silica.

Upper respiratory tract

Chronic catarrh of the middle ear with calcareous deposits that may lead to ringing in the ear and even deafness strongly suggest the use of Calc Fluor. The characteristic discharge of calcium fluoride imbalance is thick, green-yellow and lumpy.

For enlarged tonsils with plugs of mucus forming within, associated with constantly hardened glands, Calc Fluor should be considered.

Tongue

In a person with a calcium fluoride imbalance the tongue almost always has cracks or furrows, mainly in the centre. There may also be 'mapping' on the tongue, but this is more characteristic of Nat Mur.

Teeth

There is always a tendency to caries in the Calc Fluor picture, because of deficient tooth enamel. Sodium Fluoride, the form in which fluoride is added to our water systems, does not seem to help the calcium fluoride-imbalanced person, who is extremely sensitive to the form in which fluoride is presented. There may be a yellowish covering on the teeth.

The characteristic Calc Fluor lack of tissue tone may also present itself as a looseness of teeth. In severe cases teeth may be small and irregularly shaped and spaced. The teeth are also very sensitive to cold food and drink, as protective enamel is often lacking. These are good reasons to consider Calc Fluor.

Gut

When there is a loss of tissue elasticity, prolapsed conditions* can easily develop, such as hiatus hernia, bowel 'pockets' leading to irritable bowl and constipation, and internal and external haemorrhoids. Calc Fluor should be considered to help repair and stem the tendency towards these prolapsed states.

Respiratory system

Calc Fluor can be considered for croup* or any breathing problem* that is related to impairment of the inherent flexibility and elasticity of the respiratory tract. Expectoration of small lumps of green-yellow mucus will be characteristic of respiratory complaints.

Circulatory system

Loss of elasticity resulting from a calcium fluoride imbalance can promote dilation of blood vessels causing enlarged or varicose veins that at their most extreme may be prone to lesions* because they are as fragile as old rubber bands. Coldness and numbness of extremities may result from an inability of weakened or toneless peripheral veins to distribute an efficient blood supply in these areas. Chilblains may develop. Calc Fluor can often be of assistance.

As mentioned before, Calc Fluor is the prime remedy to consider for a history of haemorrhoids, which are a form of varicosity.

Female

For all forms of uterine tissue overproduction* such as fibroids and endometriosis consider Calc Fluor as the main tissue salt, usually in conjunction with Silica. When there is any overproduction of tissue, there is usually an accompanying loss of elasticity in the area, hence the need for Calc Fluor. Recurring and chronic hard nodes and indurated glands* of the breast may also be helped by this tissue salt.

Male

Calc Fluor with Silica should be considered for indurations (tissue hardening) and enlargements of the prostate.*

Urinary system

Poor tissue elasticity can manifest as insufficiently developed bladder tone in the young, or bladder weakness as a part of the aging process. In either case Calc Fluor is the key tissue salt.

Structural system

Some general Calc Fluor indications are hard swellings in the form of cysts and ganglia, enlargements of joints causing restriction of movement, and crepitation in or cracking of joints due to hardening and/or deterioration of bone surfaces. It should also be considered for fractures failing to unite (especially when Calc Phos is not indicated), and for trauma-induced 'bruised' bones. Calc Fluor may be considered for lower backache and other bone pains if they are generally worse after any cold exposure and at night, and are better with heat.

The nails may show similar indications to those calling for Calc Phos, but are more likely to have a tendency to peel or split easily.

Skin

Those needing Calc Fluor may have a tendency to fissure formation and hardening and thickening of the skin, which may include scarring that is slow to resolve. For this tendency, Calc Fluor would be used in conjunction with Silica.

Calc Fluor may be considered where premature lines and wrinkles develop if skin elasticity declines at a much faster rate than you would normally expect due to aging.

Sleep

Dreams of a disturbing nature, fearful and full of impending doom and danger are characteristic of all calcium imbalances, which by their nature affect body structure – the foundations of our being. There is often a resulting unconscious feeling of fragility and vulnerability which may find expressions in dreams.

General

Better by:

Calcium fluoride-imbalanced people and their symptoms are especially responsive to heat, warm applications, massage and rest.

Worse by:

Cold, beginning to move, and changes in weather, especially from dry to damp weather, can aggravate symptoms of the person in need of Calc Fluor.

Complementary and related salts

Calc Fluor and Silica work synergistically to help in bone disorders and indurated (hardened) infiltrations and overproductions of tissue in the body.

Kali Phos is related to Calc Fluor in that it helps to improve mental tenacity and tone. It is the first tissue salt to consider for mental fatigue, before Calc Fluor and Silica.

Supportive measures

Exercising maintains suppleness and increases flexibility and tone: all extremely important for the calcium fluoride-imbalanced person. A moderate daily routine, preferably of short but frequent sessions, would enhance well-being.

A diet full of fibre is very important to keep things toned internally for those with a calcium fluoride imbalance.

Diet

Buckwheat and rye bread, pumpkin, cabbage, onions, grapes, oranges and lemons (especially the pith which is also rich in bioflavonoids), are all rich in calcium fluoride. The substances known as bioflavonoids act synergistically with the mineral. There are two types of fluorides: sodium fluoride which is added to drinking water is NOT the same as calcium fluoride, the form used by the body. Herbs rich in calcium fluoride are chickweed, hamamelis (witch hazel) and rue.

Flower essences

Clematis (Bach), Sundew (Aus Bush) and Lemon (FES) can help to remedy the characteristic lack of mental tone and 'grounded' focus of calcium fluoride imbalance. Trillium (FES) can help with fear of lack, or 'poverty consciousness' underlying fears of financial ruin. Willow (Bach) may help those who lack the mental and emotional resilience to face the 'trials and tribulations' of life, and who may reflect this in a body that is also lacking resilience and elasticity.

Related disciplines

Iridology

In the iris, first evidence of a calcium fluoride imbalance is displayed in a dilated nerve wreath showing a tendency to bowl 'pockets'. Radii solaris are an indication that the gut lining is leaking toxins back into the tissues of the body. The integrity of the gut wall has become compromised through lack of elasticity, tone and flexibility.

Astrology

Lack of tone is often a physical feature of the Cancerian constitution. Those with a strong Cancerian signature may, like their body tissues, sometimes lack the resilience to spring back in a vital way after life's trials. Calc Fluor may be of assistance to these natures, as it can be for anyone whose strong water element causes a tendency to unclear definition of mental, emotional and physical boundaries.

Keywords

Elasticity, flexibility, resilience, tone.

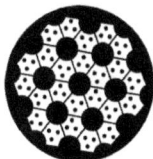

Calc Phos

Calcium phosphate

Calcium phosphate is found in bones, teeth, connective tissue, blood corpuscles and gastric juice. It is a basic structural component in the body. It is also an essential constituent of every bodily tissue or fluid apart from connective tissue. It plays a significant role in the entire nutritional process from digestion through to cell and tissue growth and energy expenditure.

Body type

People especially sensitive to Calc Phos, in other words those with a long-standing imbalance related to its crude mineral counterpart, are tall, thin and rapidly growing individuals who are easily fatigued. They may look pale and be very cold sensitive due to deficient circulation. Calc Phos is particularly beneficial during phases of rapid tissue growth such as those experienced by children and pregnant women.

Mind

If there is an imbalance or deficiency of calcium phosphate in the brain cells their efficiency will be impaired. Confidence in mental receptivity and agility declines. As a result, especially in children, fears of failure and the humiliation that results from being unable to respond intelligently may cause avoidance of anything that might provide the slightest challenge. They simply do not try for fear of failure, and may appear obstinate as a result. Other consequences of calcium phosphate deficiency in children are poor comprehension, concentration and memory, anxiety over trivia, tearfulness and irritability. For these symptoms in an adult, however, think of Kali Phos.

Head

Headaches with accompanying feelings of coldness and numbness in the head are characteristic of the person in need of Calc Phos. So too the headaches that come on directly after exposure to cold conditions. It can be especially useful for headaches of childhood, puberty or pregnancy, if for no other reason than that these are times when calcium phosphate is in great demand in the body.

Eyes

For oversensitivity to light and for spasmodic affections of the eye, consider Calc Phos in conjunction with, or after Mag Phos.

Ears

For any earache* that occurs after exposure to cold consider Calc Phos. The tissue salt is almost certainly required by children suffering from chronic catarrh of the ear and persistent enlarged lymph glands in the neck concurrently. Calc Phos, along with other tissue salts, is indicated for the majority of chronic ailments in children.

Upper respiratory tract

The characteristic Cal Phos nasal catarrh is albuminous and sometimes streaked with blood.

Tonsils and adenoids* are commonly enlarged in children requiring Calc Phos. The presence of a post-nasal drip can contribute to a constant hoarseness and the need to hawk. Frequent ear, nose and throat infections* in children always signal a need for Calc Phos.

Teeth

Efficient and normal dental development as with all structural development of the body is dependent on the proper assimilation and use of calcium phosphate. In children, problems with the assimilation will show in a tendency to delayed dentition and complaints during teething such as a tendency to nasal catarrh or proneness to infection.

Rapid and widespread decay in teeth will be the trend if calcium phosphate is in imbalance, but think of Calc Fluor too. Gums may become painful, inflamed or pale.

Gut

Calc Phos can assist with inefficient food absorption and poor appetite, especially in children. It is also very helpful in cases of heartburn, flatulence and bloating, especially when given with Nat Phos, Mag Phos, and often Nat Sulph.

Another possible indication for Calc Phos is constant craving for savoury and salty foods, although Nat Mur is even more likely to have this symptom. Always consider Calc Phos in conjunction with Mag Phos for colic or any other spasmodic or irritable affliction of the gastrointestinal tract.

Respiratory system

Any person prone to recurrent or chronic respiratory infections* will almost certainly benefit from taking Calc Phos over an extended period. Symptoms aggravated by exposure to cold air are a clear indication for its use. Calc Phos may be of great benefit during convalescence after seriously incapacitating respiratory ailments.*

Circulatory system

If there is poor circulation indicated by cold or numb extremities, perhaps with accompanying chilblains, you would be wise to consider Calc Phos. Circulatory cramps, especially when they begin or intensify in cold conditions can also be a strong indication.

Female

Painful menstrual cramping* can be characteristic of calcium phosphate imbalance, especially when it occurs in pubescent or rapidly growing females. Always consider Calc Phos in conjunction with Mag Phos for any type of spasm or cramping. Calc Phos is essential during pregnancy (once again consider Mag Phos also) when demands for calcium during new growth are so great.

Urinary system

For bed-wetting associated with fearful dreams and night terrors consider Calc Phos, usually in conjunction with other remedies, especially flower essences.

Bladder and kidney stones* that are mainly composed of calcium compounds indicate an imbalance in the distribution of calcium in the body. Taking Calc Phos often helps. An over acid system encourages the development of deposits in the body, and Nat Phos will often help in such a case.

Structural system

For all rheumatic pains and numbness in bones and muscles that are worse for any exposure to cold, Calc Phos must be considered. Growing pains in the bones, shin soreness and fractured bones that are slow to heal are all strong indications for Calc Phos. Also for all degrees of osteoporosis* Calc Phos presents natural calcium in an easily assimilated form that can therefore be properly utilised by an ageing metabolism. This has a chain-reaction effect in the body in that it encourages more efficient uptake of calcium from foodstuffs as well. All tissue salts seem to share this ability to pass these effects along.

Calc Phos indications in the nails are the appearance of white flecks and/or marked brittleness. Brittleness can also be seen in those needing Silica.

Skin

With a calcium deficiency the complexion of the skin can become pale and unhealthy looking. After Kali Mur, Calc Phos should be considered as the next most important tissue salt for warts (and for nasal, rectal and uterine polyps*). Best results will be gained if the remedy is given over a long period. The general integrity of the skin is dependent on proper utilisation of calcium in the body.

Sleep

Vivid, fearful and disturbing dreams in children can be an indication for Calc Phos. (Consider also the use of flower essences.) Obviously one must also look for underlying causes*

General

Better by:

Those with a calcium phosphate imbalance feel better in themselves and in their symptoms after rest, lying down ('taking the weight off' a weak body structure) and with warmth.

Worse by:

Any form of COLD, prolonged motion without a break, and any change in the weather but especially from warmer to cold weather. Also, worse during dentition and other times of rapid physical growth.

Complementary and related salts

Mag Phos and Calc Phos act synergistically as natural anti-spasmodics, digestive aids and as structural building materials in the body.

Calc Phos supports Ferrum Phos in cases of circulatory weakness.

Calc Phos relates to Silica in the body's structural development. Calcium phosphate can be seen as nature's raw building material while Silica acts as nature's 'sculptor' by governing the proper deposition and distribution of calcium in the body.

Supportive measures

A healthy lifestyle that maintains enough sleep and good nutrition is absolutely essential for a person with a need for assistance in the proper utilisation of calcium.

Exercise is useful to encourage better consolidation of calcium phosphate in bones, strengthening the body's structural components. Exercise also helps to mobilise the sluggish circulation.

'Prepare yourself to take some risks in life'.

Diet

Good sources of calcium are green leafy vegetables, carrots, lentils, eggs, whole grains, many of the berry fruits, figs, plumbs, meat and dairy products. Herbs rich in calcium phosphate are comfrey root, horsetail, slippery elm, chamomile, pulsatilla, cramp bark.

Flower essences

Mimulus (Bach) can assist with known fears, while Garlic and St John's Wort (both FES) and Aspen (Bach) can help with deeper feelings of uneasiness, fragility and vulnerability. Crab Apple (Bach) may also be considered when there is an obsession about bodily ailments, and Cherry Plum (Bach) helps to counteract the fear of being out of control.

Related disciplines
Iridology

The iris of those who will most benefit from Calc Phos is of an open, 'honeycomb' structure. This signifies that relatively speaking the bodies of these people need more support in structural development and tissue regeneration. Also the presence of nerve or spasm rings may indicate a need for Calc Phos in conjunction with Mag Phos.

Astrology

Calc Phos relates strongly to the Capricornian need to build a positive attitude because of the importance in bone nutrition as the 'building material' of the body, and as a stabiliser of the nervous system. It also relates to Saturnian issues of structuring and restructuring of our lives in order to feel better supported and safer.

Keywords

Cell builder, raw material, general tonic, growth supporter.

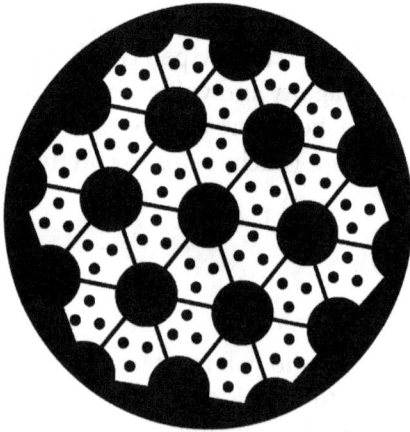

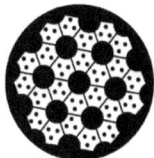

Calc Sulph

Calcium sulphate

Calcium sulphate is found in the epithelial cells of the skin, in blood and bile from the liver. It helps destroy and rid the body of worn out or unfit red blood cells. If there is a deficiency of calcium sulphate, an oversupply of 'worn out' or inefficient blood cells may accumulate, resulting in abnormal discharges from wounds, and infections that persist too long. In other words a general state of slow healing and inhibited elimination may arise.

Mind

If the bloodstream is effectively made 'toxic' by accumulated dysfunctional blood cells the mind can become correspondingly 'toxic'. For the person in need of Calc Sulph this manifests as moodiness, irritability and an overactive, worried and cluttered mind, especially at night when sleep is sought. The anxiety and ungrounded fears generally characteristic of calcium imbalances may surface.

Head

Frontal headaches with nausea can develop, related to a 'toxic' blood supply to the area. Dandruff, pustular acne and in extreme cases, yellow, discharging crusts* can appear on the scalp.

Face

Pimples that come to a pustular head, and other pustular conditions of the facial skin are common in the person who can benefit from Calc Sulph. A tendency to sensitive pimples under the beard or resulting from shaving also responds well.

Eyes

Abscess or inflammation of the eye with a characteristic persistent, thick yellow discharge is a strong indication for Calc Sulph.

Ears

Catarrhal deafness, especially with honey-yellow discharge* from the middle ear may warrant the use of Calc Sulph. (Consider Kali Sulph also.) Continual production of dark wax from the ear may also be indicative of the need for this tissue salt. Any relentless discharge from any area of the body* is good reason to consider the use of Calc Sulph.

Upper respiratory tract

A thick yellow discharge from the nose, sometimes streaked with blood is characteristic of Calc Sulph, but since Kali Sulph shares this symptom, check the wider symptom-picture for accurate prescription. Recurring sore and infected throat with a yellow, pustular discharge* also indicates a need for Calc Sulph.

Tongue

Typical indications for selection of Calc Sulph are a clay-coloured coating on the tongue, often with a yellow-coated base.

Teeth

Gums are often sore and prone to pustular ulceration, and may bleed easily on brushing.

Gut

Food cravings of those in need of tissue salts containing calcium all tend towards the savoury or sour. A persistent, discharging anal abscess associated with fistula* is a very strong indication for Calc Sulph, but don't disregard Silica.

Respiratory system

The Calc Sulph cough produces thick, lumpy, yellow expectoration.* (So does Kali Sulph.) It is often useful for the last stage of a chest infection with a persistent catarrh of this type.

Male

Calc Sulph is indicated for a characteristic, non-resolving and yellowish pustular discharge from the penis.*

Tissues

Calc Sulph aids in problems where there is a persistent discharge from deep within connective tissue, which is failing to resolve,* i.e. it is unable to heal. This tissue salt helps resolve the suppuration process, limiting the discharge of pus and hastening healing. Silica is more appropriate if it is necessary to promote suppuration in order to rapidly bring the healing process to maturity and then resolution.

Skin

Acne that comes to a pustular head, or any other 'toxic' expression at the skin level is often related to calcium sulphate imbalance. Boils, eczema and herpetic eruptions with the typical associated yellow discharge (see also Kali Sulph) can often benefit from Calc Sulph supplementation. Cuts, wounds, sores and ulcers that suppurate easily and are SLOW TO HEAL are usually indicative of a need for this salt.

Sleep

The person in need of Calc Sulph may suffer sleeplessness due to a mind that is made 'toxic' by relentless, recurring thoughts as a result of a toxic blood supply to the head.

General

Better by

Those in need of Calc Sulph always feel much better in open, fresh air.

Worse by

The individual feels worse in general and so do particular symptoms, in damp conditions or wet weather. Becoming overheated often aggravates symptoms also.

Complementary and related salts

Indications for prescription of Silica and Calc Sulph for chronic or recurring discharges from any part of the body are closely related. For best results it is wise to differentiate between the two on the basis of other symptoms.

It is also difficult to differentiate between symptoms calling for Kali Sulph and those requiring Calc Sulph in chronic or advanced stages of infection or disease. Again, overall symptoms can provide the key.

Supportive measures

Aerobic exercise encourages elimination through the lungs and the sweating skin and is therefore very beneficial. Elimination diets and even moderate fasting under the guidance of a health professional will assist in cleansing of the body.

'Emotional cleansing' or developing better ways of expressing what 'gets under your skin' will assist detoxification at levels other than the physical. As well as addressing these more subtle dimensions Calc Sulph can finish off the job by assisting in the cleansing of the physical body – our earthly waste-disposal avenue!

Diet

Onions, garlic and leeks are great sources of calcium sulphate. So are asparagus and other greens, and also radishes, watercress, cauliflower, figs and prunes.

Herbs rich in calcium sulphate are sarsaparilla, nettle, wormwood, horehound, red clover.

Flower essences

Willow and Chicory (Bach) should be considered for resentment and negative reactivity that becomes 'toxic' on an emotional level and which eventually manifests as physical toxicity. Trillium (FES) is a balancer of the basic human energy centre, the survival or base chakra, which governs organs and tissues especially important in the elimination of toxic waste from the body. Crab Apple (Bach) and Bottle Brush *(Aus Bush) also have a special role in cleansing at all levels.

Related disciplines

Iridology

Calc Sulph's under-active skin metabolism is most likely to show up in the iris as a dark scurf rim. This indication is shared with both Silica and Kali Sulph. Signs of heavy lymphatic congestion are usually also present.

Astrology

Scorpio natures are prone to becoming 'toxic' on an emotional level if their expression of emotional intensity (and creativity) is inhibited. This will eventually be reflected in a breakdown in effective physical 'expression' or elimination from the body. For this reason Scorpio is more prone to toxaemia than any other sign, and can therefore often be helped by Calc Sulp's eliminatory encouragement.

Keywords

Blood-purifier, resolves suppuration, dissolves discharge.

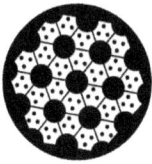

Mag Phos

Magnesium phosphate

Magnesium phosphate is a constituent of muscles, nerves, bone, brain, spine, sperm, teeth and blood corpuscles. It acts as an ANTI-SPASMODIC and its action is chiefly confined to the delicate white nerve-fibres, combining with albumin and water to form the fluid that nourishes them. Magnesium phosphate soothes and nurtures the nervous system.

Body type

Mag Phos is useful for anyone who suffers from muscular tension, bit it is particularly helpful for those of a thin and wiry build with rigid muscle formation, who burn up their body fat in nervous activity.

Mind

There is often an inability to think clearly because the mind is cluttered. Just as the muscles remain in a tense state of 'readiness' so the mind remains correspondingly alert and ready to respond. Mag Phos, in allowing the body to relax, also assists the mind to attain calm more easily. If physical tension persists, the overactive mind can become tired, depleted and depressed so that there is an indisposition to any type of mental work. In this case, Kali Phos is also indicated.

Head

Headaches of a sharp, shooting, darting, stabbing nature, or intermittent and neuralgic pains which are RELIEVED BY WARM APPLICATION are characteristic of magnesium phosphate imbalance. Nervous tension-induced headache with a tight band-like feeling around the head is another strong indication. There may be extreme sensitivity to light touch, while warmth created by the firm friction of massage brings relief.

Face

Facial neuralgic pains* that are decidedly worse for any touch or coldness and commonly worse on the right side are quite definite indications for the therapeutic use of Mag Phos.

Eyes

Magnesium phosphate imbalance may affect vision.* Blurred vision is common, as are colours, sparks, flashes, often associated with migraine. Muscular tension can also result in abnormal behaviour of the pupil, affecting its ability to control the amount of light received by the internal eye. Oversensitivity to bright light (photophobia) may develop as a result.

Neuralgia and a nagging twitching of the eyelid often respond well to Mag Phos.

Ears

Mag Phos will be among remedies for deafness resulting from damaged or tension-affected auditory nerves,* because of its nutrient-providing and anti-spasmodic qualities. Sharp neuralgic* pains in and around the ear, stress-induced ringing in the ear and earache* all suggest the need for Mag Phos.

Upper respiratory tract

Loss or perversion of the sense of smell, especially without significant production of catarrh can be a good indication for Mag Phos. (Consider Kali Phos also.)

It is the prime remedy for spasmodic constriction and closing of the throat – Globus Hystericus.* Mag Phos is useful in any mucous membrane spasm,* whether of the respiratory or digestive tract.

Consider Mag Phos in conjunction with other tissue salts in all thyroid-related problems.*

Teeth

When there is a need for Mag Phos, teeth are commonly ultra-sensitive to cold and touch. There may be severe PAIN in decayed or filled teeth, accompanied by spasmodic, sharp, shooting nerve pains.* All Mag Phos pains are better for hot applications.

Complaints associated with teething, especially neuralgic pains, often respond well to Mag Phos. (Consider Calc Phos and Ferrum Phos also.)

Gut

Hiccough, heartburn (always use Nat Phos as well), griping pains, spasms and cramps relieved by warmth and bending over double are all strong indications for Mag Phos. Mag Phos will almost always help flatulent Colic where pain forces the person to bend double and is temporarily relieved by massage, warmth, pressure, and expulsion of gas. Bloating of the abdomen (consider also Nat Sulph), and stress-related irritable bowl* are strong indications for Mag Phos.

Consider Mag Phos for sugar addiction to help reduce craving. Kali Sulph may also be helpful.

Respiratory system

Bronchial spasm causing chest or breathing constriction always indicates a need for Mag Phos,* among other remedies.

Circulatory system

Mag Phos should be prominent among tissue salts considered for cases of constriction or spasm of blood vessels, and for nervous palpitation of the heart.*

Female

Mag Phos is a key tissue salt for helping ease general menstrual pain and colic, premenstrual pain and tension, and cramping pain associated with the discharge of dark clots.* It is equally useful for pain and cramping associated with ovulation.*

Male

Mag Phos can assist in cases of premature ejaculation and other tension-related sexual problems.*

Urinary system

Constant urging with incomplete urination in adults,* or nervous, spasmodic urine retention during the day and then nocturnal enuresis in children are all good indications for the use of Mag Phos. This remedy should also be considered in the treatment of bladder stones and gravel.* It can help ease painful spasm usually associated with these conditions and assist in dissolving and breaking down the stones, especially when calcium is their major constituent. (Use in conjunction with Silica.) Mag Phos plays a very important role in calcium phosphate metabolism.

Structural system

Those for whom Mag Phos is useful often suffer from characteristic muscular cramps and/or sharp shooting pains, especially in the middle back. Other nervous symptoms such as trembling hands are common.

The nails of a person with a constitutional need for magnesium often have a broad base and are short relative to their width. They may have fine vertical ridging. (This symptom also indicates a need for Silica.) Otherwise nails can show similar characteristics to those that indicate a need for Calc Phos.

Skin

For stress-related skin ailments Mag Phos, along with Kali Phos among others, is always useful.

Sleep

Twitching of the limbs just prior to sleep, or immediately after falling asleep are common indications for the use of Mag Phos. Vivid, active and often sleep-disrupting dreams often follow.

General

Better by:

All Mag Phos-related symptoms are improved by HEAT, massage and pressure. Many digestive symptoms feel better while bending double.

Worse by:

An imbalance in magnesium phosphate can often be reflected in health problems that are worse on the right side of the body, although this is not invariable. Cold in all forms and light touch aggravates symptoms, as does glare with regard to eye symptoms. Mag Phos is essential for the nervous after-effects of alcohol abuse.

Complementary and related salts

Mag Phos combines well with and is complemented by Calc Phos for any type of muscular spasm.

It is also given frequently with Kali Phos for the effects of stress and nervous exhaustion.

Mag Phos and Silica both assist in the proper structural deployment of calcium in the body.

Supportive measures

Relaxation and mindfulness practices will benefit the person in need of Mag Phos. So will yoga, tai chi and the gentle and relaxing movement of walking or swimming. Massage can be profoundly helpful.

A lifestyle with a balance of work, rest and play is essential. Remember 'Thy will be done', not necessarily 'My will be done', so relax and learn just to let life happen sometimes!

Diet

Peas, lettuce and other green leafy vegetables; almonds, walnuts, oats, citrus fruits and bananas, plums, apples and bonemeal are good sources of magnesium phosphate. Please note that the B vitamins, especially vitamin B6, act synergistically with magnesium in the body.

Herbs that are rich in magnesium phosphate are chamomile, cramp bark, gelsemium, comfrey, dill, the mints, passionflower, skullcap and valerian.

Flower essences

Dandelion (FES) is excellent for the tense, overzealous person. Vervain (Bach) is useful for a similar type of person who tries too hard or is over-enthusiastic about a cause and as a result becomes tense and drained of energy. Impatiens (Bach) helps with just what its name suggests and the nervous tension that so often results.

Related disciplines
Iridology

Strong indication in the iris of a need for Mag Phos comes in the form of a contracted nerve wreath, or one that is irregular, showing many inward deviations. Other indications are the presence of lightly coloured nerve or cramp rings.

Astrology

Leo natures are prone to excess, and to pushing themselves to get 'out there' to meet the world head on. As a result they can carry much nervous tension in the body and easily become exhausted. Mag Phos can also help in the opposite circumstance, when a person has difficulty accessing the vital, fiery and creative energies associated with Leo and Mars, precipitating much frustration and hence inner tension.

Keywords

Nerve and muscular relaxant and nutrient; relieves nerve pain.

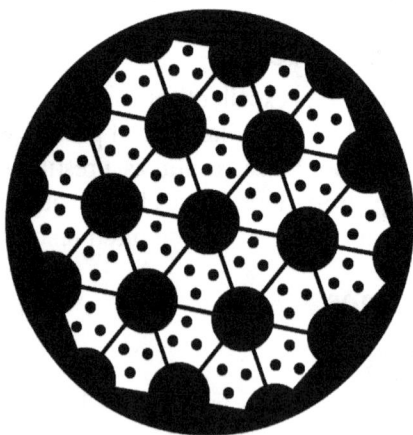

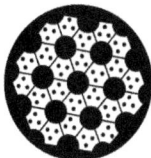

Silica

Silica

In the biosphere, Silica is mainly found in the vegetable kingdom and in the bodies of vertebrates, creatures with spinal columns. Among animals the more structured an organism is, the more it seems to need this mineral. Silica is present in blood, bile, skin, hair, nails, connective tissue, bones, nerve sheaths and mucous membranes. It plays an essential role in proper formation and maintenance of connective tissue, acting like a cellular 'cement' which strongly influences the development of the body-structure.

Body type

The constitution with a deep-seated Silica imbalance has sometimes been described as a body 'without backbone', a person lacking moral 'grit', or a 'piston with no rod'. People who will respond in the most profound way to Silica are usually thin, weak and demineralised, and are either poor eaters or have a digestive system lacking in the ability to effectively assimilate nutrients. They are always very cold sensitive.

Children can be sickly in the extreme, with large abdomens and a large head in proportion to their underweight limbs. Adults are often nervous, intelligent types who are prone to infection.

Mind

Those in need of Silica are often quick-minded but shy and they experience great anticipatory anxiety before occasions when they must display their mental powers; at worst they can be hypersensitive, nervous, irritable and anxious. This affects their ability to concentrate and they may mentally tire easily. (Consider Kali Phos also.) In response to this anxiety, children may appear obstinate, timid or shy, whilst adults may develop very fixed ideas and become set in ways that are familiar and safe, staying in their 'comfort zone'. This approach may in fact turn out to be a strength, giving the ability to endure and to remain absolutely loyal to a successful approach to studies, business or life. People needing Silica may be slow developers, but once they start achieving their goals there is no looking back.

Head

Silica is an extremely important nutrient for hair and nails, and the tissue salt should be considered whenever any problem challenges the integrity of these formations, as in cases of falling hair or splitting nails.

A characteristic Silica headache begins in the occiput and extends over the head, settling over the eye (often the right eye). Some relief is obtained by application of warmth and/or wrapping up the head, applying some pressure. The pain is worse with any noise, light or mental exertion. Suppression of a persistent or bad-smelling foot-sweat can sometimes cause a tendency to headaches, when toxins unable to find an outlet via sweating must be recycled throughout the body. Silica can reverse this process, initially lessening headaches and eventually moderating foot-sweats as the body's eliminatory organs (especially the kidneys) are encouraged to do their job more efficiently.

Face

If there is acne it is often 'blind' and with a tendency to linger, sometimes culminating in scarring. Subcutaneous (just below the skin) lumps and nodules are a common indication for Silica, whose 'centrifugal' action in the body has the ability to bring these accumulations 'out' to maturity so that they may be quickly resolved.

Minor cracking of the skin may also be present. (Consider Calc Fluor also.)

Eyes

STYES on the eyelids are a classical indication for the use of Silica, especially if they are recurring. Styes are a very clear example of 'blind' eruptions characteristic of Silica imbalance. There is often a thick, yellow-green discharge associated with any eye problems.

Silica is prescribed in conjunction with Calc Fluor for cataract,* or any hardening and overproduction of tissue.

Silica is indicated if Mag Phos has failed to adequately relieve photophobia.*

Ears

For oversensitivity to noise, or for its opposite in the form of dulled hearing resulting from swelling and catarrh of the Eustachian tubes,* especially with a discharge of a thick, yellow-green matter,

Silica should be strongly considered. Remember that Silica is invariably required for any chronic, recurring catarrhal infection,* including of the ears, in children.

Throat

Silica is needed where there is slow-to-heal, recurring suppuration (pus formation) of the tonsils.*

Characteristic of the body's need for Silica is the following pattern of a struggling immune system. An initial dis-ease is felt as a sore throat which quickly re-manifests as a nasal discharge and then rapidly descends to lodge itself in the chest.* In other words, the first defence of tonsils and nasal mucous membranes fails to protect long enough to allow the rest of the body time to acquire general natural immunity to the infection. This leaves vital organs such as the bronchioles and lungs vulnerable to easy infiltration by infection, weakening the whole organism and leaving the body open to a repetition of the cycle.

Teeth

When there is a deep-seated and persistent toothache,* especially if Mag Phos fails to give satisfactory relief, Silica is indicated.

A root abscess* that can find no avenue of escape for its pustular contents requires Silica. However if a discharge is already established, Calc Sulph may be more appropriate.*

Gut

The need for Silica is classically displayed in the thin child with a large abdomen, who is unable to properly assimilate nutrients. Constipation is very common, with a characteristic 'bashful' stool, i.e. the stool recedes after being partly expelled. Silica warrants strong consideration when using tissue salts to treat anal fissures* (also consider Calc Fluor), and fistulas* (Calc Sulph may be useful also).

Respiratory system

As mentioned earlier, infections requiring Silica often start in the throat, ascend to the nose, then quickly settle in the chest* and are slow to resolve. This pattern tends to repeat, and infection is most likely accompanied by a persistent, thick yellow-green and lumpy expectoration.

Circulatory system

People in need of Silica are very chilly and cold-sensitive. Their feet may sweat but at the same time feel very cold.

Female

Premenstrual constipation is common to many women, but it is even more common in those that may benefit from taking Silica. The cold-sensitivity experienced by those needing this tissue salt is often heightened premenstrually and during menses.

Structural system

Silica supports Calc Fluor in strengthening and recovery of weak or damaged tendons, ligaments and spinal discs.* It assists in all structural problems of the body and in particular, brittle nails and hair, or nails that display ridging. Ingrown toenails* and ingrowing hairs, or any other body structure exhibiting an imbalance in calcium metabolism all indicate a need for Silica.

Tissues

Silica helps promote suppuration when pustular material is confined and unable to find a way of evacuation from the body.* It resolves suppuration by bringing the process to maturity. Calc Sulph, on the other hand, is useful for persistent, unconfined suppuration,* bringing it to its proper completion. Silica can also be used to prevent further suppuration if there is a pattern of recurrence. In this situation it is best taken in the quiescent stage between reoccurrences.

For long-standing fungal growths affecting toenails and fingernails, Silica and/or Kali Sulph should be strongly considered.

Skin

Long-term Silica imbalance may present as generally poor skin that is slow to heal and has a tendency to scarring. Nails and hair are also of a poor quality. Acne, boils and subcutaneous cysts commonly occur. Fetid sweats, especially of the feet, are common. The skin of fingers may become dry and cracked, particularly in times of nervous stress.

Because of its 'centrifugal action' in the body, Silica should always be considered to help promote expulsion of foreign bodies from the tissues,* e.g. when there is some concern that glass or splinters may have remained lodged in a wound after treatment.

Sleep

When Mag Phos fails to improve the tendency to jerking and twitching of limbs just prior to and during first sleep, Silica may be a useful second choice.

General

Better by:

The person who requires Silica has symptoms that feel better from exposure to all forms of WARMTH. General well-being improves under warm conditions, and in summer.

Worse by:

COLD and especially cold air will aggravate symptoms and decrease general well-being. Symptoms may be most intense at night.

People needing Silica are more sensitive to their environment than others. This can even extend to an uncomfortable and heightened awareness of moon phases, especially the FULL MOON. The mind may be uncontrollably active at this time.

Complementary and related salts

Calc Fluor complements the action of Silica in cases of structural and tissue overproduction, induration and deformity.

Silica helps ensure the proper employment and distribution of calcium and magnesium (see Calc Phos and Mag Phos) in the body, especially in times of rapid growth and when there are digestive disturbances.

Calc Sulph is related to Silica through its influence on suppurative processes, but their actions are different – see above, 'Tissues'.

In nervous complaints when Mag Phos fails to have its usual effect, Silica should always be considered as an adjunct or alternative.

Supportive measures

The 'brittleness' of those needing Silica can be helped by regular exercise that focuses on strengthening and maintaining flexibility in the body's pivoting, structural apparatus. Like those needing Calc Fluor they will benefit by working on the elasticity of the body, and like Calc Phos people they will benefit by working on bodily strength and endurance. Tai chi and swimming are ways to help more fluidity of movement, and ultimately fluidity of approach to life.

Don't be afraid to try a whole new approach sometimes, so that when change comes by itself, it won't be such a shock!

Diet

Silica is found in celery, carrots, oats, rye, rice and all other cereals, the skin and fibre (pith) of fruit and vegetables, in drinking water and especially in the herb horsetail (equisetum). Other herbs containing this mineral are chicory, dandelion and pulsatilla.

Flower essences

The centrifugal action of Silica on a physical level has its analogy in the centrifugal action of Agrimony (Bach) on an emotional level, i.e. Agrimony helps to externalise feelings that have become painful by being locked inside. Also consider Violet (FES) for that sensitive soul who shies away from sharing feelings and valuable insights about the world.

Californian Poppy (FES) can help with overactivity and nervous scattering of energies in the 'restlessly seeking' individual.

Related disciplines

Iridology

A need for Silica is often expressed in the iris in a way similar to that for Mag Phos: a characteristic contracted nerve wreath with a relatively toxic bowel indication. The iris structure or 'texture' may be surprisingly good and clear, with a contrasting darker, scurf rim indicating under-active skin.

Astrology

Silica can be especially supportive and strengthening to the Sagittarian who has become nervously depleted through overactivity and scattering of fiery personal energies. It may also be useful when there is an inability to express the fire element.

Keywords

Eliminates toxins, matures and prevents recurrence of suppuration, organises and reorganises calcium metabolism.

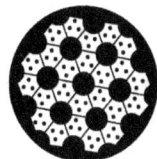

Ferrum Phos

Iron phosphate

Iron is found in the haemoglobin of blood, responsible for carrying oxygen to all parts of the body. Oxygen of course is essential for sustaining life, so you could say that iron helps 'breathe life' into tissues and cells, especially when they become vulnerable to invasion by organisms of a viral nature. That is why Ferrum Phos is the tissue salt to consider at the first sign of any infection or inflammation. In fact it is the first tissue salt to consider for any ailment that ends its medical name in 'itis' as this implies an inflammatory condition.

Iron also gives strength to the circular walls of blood vessels, especially arteries which are the bulk distributors of iron in the form of oxygen-rich blood to body-tissues and cells. The organic basis of every cell is albumin, which also contains iron.

Body type

The classic picture of someone who has been deficient in iron phosphate for a long time is the tired, pale and anaemic-looking child or adolescent who is very prone to infection. There is often a tendency to nose-bleed. In both children and adults, the face may flush easily, and this redness is in contrast to their normally pale complexion. In the more mature person a ruddy, florid complexion may develop.

Often the upper body is hot in contrast to cold lower parts, e.g. the face may become hot and red while the feet are cold.

Mind

During over-heated conditions of the body, for example fever, the mental state can fluctuate between complete indifference or listlessness, and IRRITABILITY. In conditions of long-term iron deficiency, the brain may experience oxygen deprivation, resulting in forgetfulness, vagueness and states of dizziness and faintness. Consider the overall picture in order to differentiate between the need for Kali Phos and Ferrum Phos.

Head

All the usual symptoms associated with fever, ranging from dizziness to delirium, warrant the use of Ferrum Phos. For the first stage of any head cold with either a clear nasal discharge or none at all, it is the prime tissue salt. Consider Ferrum Phos plus the glandular remedies Kali Mur and Nat Mur for hot flushes* associated with menopause.

Face

As mentioned earlier, a pale, anaemic complexion that flushes red easily is a good indication for Ferrum Phos. A ruddy, florid complexion may develop as a result of long-term deficiency or declining availability of iron.

Eyes

Red, bloodshot, inflamed eyes, especially when associated with burning sensations often respond well to Ferrum Phos. A sensation of grains of sand lodged under the eyelids, as in the initial stages of conjunctivitis,* is another good indication for the use of Ferrum Phos.

Ears

For the inflamed, burning, throbbing and/or red ear,* particularly as a result of exposure to cold or wet conditions, Ferrum Phos is strongly indicated. Its use is a good first response to ear infections* of children, helping to resolve them quickly. Administer Ferrum Phos as often as every ten minutes in such a case.

Upper respiratory tract

Spontaneous nosebleeds or bright blood from any outlet* for that matter are indications for Ferrum Phos. So is the dry, hot beginning or initial clear catarrh of head colds. If an inflamed throat is red and dry* without any exudation, and there is accompanying thirst, Ferrum Phos should help. There may also be loss of voice, or hoarseness.

Tongue

An indication for Ferrum Phos is a tongue that is bright red and either clear or with darker red swellings. It is useful for ulcers of a red and inflamed aspect, but for any ulcerated condition it would seldom be prescribed alone.

Teeth

Ferrum Phos is indicated for fever, heat or redness associated with teething. Remember that great demands on calcium at this time suggest Calc Phos also. For toothache* always consider a combination of Ferrum Phos and Mag Phos, among other remedies.

Gut

When Ferrum Phos is required there may be a tendency to diarrhoea and an undigested stool. This is especially the case with children and may well be associated with multiple food allergies* or intolerances.

For haemorrhoids with bright red bleeding,* use Ferrum Phos with other tissue salts indicated by the overall symptom picture.

Respiratory system

Ferrum Phos is indicated in early inflammatory stages of all infections. Use in combination with Mag Phos when there is shortness of breath associated with infection, e.g. in cases of bronchitis in young children.* For chronic problems with the integrity of mucous membranes of the respiratory tract* always consider Ferrum Phos and Kali Sulph, taken in combination over some time.

Circulatory system

Ferrum Phos is indicated when there is palpitation with rapid pulse* associated with fever or overheating. A tendency to haemorrhage,* especially nose bleeds, may be a feature of the need for Ferrum Phos. Anaemic people or those with blood insufficiencies* usually benefit from Ferrum Phos plus other selected tissue salts.

Female

When menstrual pain is caused by an inflammatory reaction,* for example when pain has been alleviated in the past by anti-inflammatory drugs, Ferrum Phos is the first tissue salt to consider, with Mag Phos in conjunction for cramping pain. These remedies would need to be taken throughout 3-6 full menstrual cycles to achieve the best results. Initially, for painful episodes during menstruation more frequent doses (up to every fifteen minutes) can be administered.

Urinary system

At the first signs of any burning or pain of cystitis,* Ferrum Phos is indicated in combination with Nat Phos which helps to make the whole system and therefore the urine more alkaline. As cystitis is an acute condition, best results will be achieved by taking salts frequently, perhaps every fifteen minutes initially.

Structural system

For any inflammation of muscles, joints, etc. whether as a result of trauma or as part of a rheumatic diathesis, Ferrum Phos is strongly indicated. Think of it as tissue salt first aid for any injury, strain or sprain,* assisting circulatory response in the affected area so that healing can progress efficiently and rapidly.

Tissues

The pre-exudative stage of any inflammation or infection is the primary indication for the use of Ferrum Phos. Think of it immediately whenever there is an active inflammatory process, local or general.*

Skin

Hyperaemia,* i.e. localised blood accumulation characterised by redness, heat and often swelling warrants the use of Ferrum Phos. It also helps reduce heat, blood accumulation, pain and throbbing of wounds, abscesses, boils etc., especially from their beginning to their peak. Ferrum Phos hastens natural healing processes to a rapid and satisfactory conclusion.

General

Better by:

General well-being as well as particular symptoms of those needing Ferrum Phos are better for cold applications to affected areas and warmth to the body as a whole, which tends to give off heat in localised areas and have difficulty retaining it overall. GENTLE exercise and motion over an extended period, warming up to everyday tasks, will help.

Worse by:

Heightened activity, excitement, demands for short intense energy bursts aggravate all symptoms and lessen the general well-being of those needing Ferrum Phos. There is usually an aggravation even from passive overheating, and at night.

Complementary and related salts

Kali Mur complements Ferrum Phos as an immune regulator and mucous membrane normaliser, and as a natural anti-inflammatory. Kali Sulph may be an alternative to Ferrum Phos, particularly in chronic conditions where discharges are consistently yellow or yellow-green.

Kali Sulph relates to Ferrum Phos in its ability to enhance oxygenation of blood cells and therefore tissues, especially of the skin and mucous membranes of the respiratory tract.

Supportive measures

Moderate aerobic activity that gently assists blood flow will improve well-being, e.g. walking, swimming, yoga and tai chi. Those needing Ferrum Phos will benefit by learning to consolidate their energies and curb an over-sympathetic nature.

In the words of the personal growth guru's favourite cliché, 'Commit yourself to Life'.

Diet

Foods rich in iron are spinach, lettuce, parsley, liver, red meat, lentils, radishes, celery, horseradish, strawberries, apples, kelp, onions, almonds, walnuts and sesame seeds (tahini). Nettle and yarrow are two herbs particularly rich in iron. The taking of Ferrum Phos improves the body's uptake and assimilation of iron from these foods.

Flower essences

If there is an underlying fear of full involvement in or commitment to life which expresses itself somatically in low blood pressure or red blood deficiency,* consider Wild Rose (Bach) to restore enthusiasm and passion for life, or Rock Rose (Bach) to overcome the sheer terror of 'being here' on Earth. For more acute inflammatory responses consider essences of red flowers, especially Indian Pink, Scarlet Monkeyflower and Black Eyed Susan (all FES) which address underlying inflammatory emotional and mental responses to life. Finally, Waratah (Aus Bush) is also excellent to help with fear that prevents being fully grounded in the present and taking on life's challenges.

Related disciplines

Iridology

Areas of the iris displaying a lightened or white 'flaring' appearance signify inflammation and congestion and therefore a need for Ferrum Phos. In cases of chronic iron deficiency you may find a faded or light blue scurf rim.

Astrology

Piscean natures may suffer from scattered life energies and an inability to really focus in the 'here and now'. Like all water signs, they can be easily swayed and psychically influenced or drained, leaving them vulnerable to emotional and therefore physical imbalances. Ferrum Phos can help strengthen the very ground of being, through the experience of firmly planted feet, well-supplied with blood, which allow Piscean natures to 'stand up for themselves' independently.

Keywords

First stage of infection; inflammation resolver (general and local), 'cooler' of RED and overheated conditions.

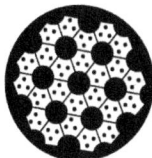

Kali Mur

Potassium chloride

Potassium chloride unites with albumin to form fibrin which is found in every tissue of the body except bones. When there is an imbalance of this mineral, it causes the release of albumin, creating a thick, white, sticky secretion that is difficult to expel. This discharge, mainly from mucous membranes and serous membranes, often follows an oedematous (fluid retentive) stage indicating the need for Ferrum Phos: Kali Mur corresponds to the SECOND STAGE OF INFLAMMATION.

Body type

Those needing Kali Mur often have chronic glandular problems, commonly manifesting in a congested lymphatic system. The lymphatic system is like the body's rubbish disposal system and if it becomes 'clogged' infection will tend to appear to feed off resultant stagnant waste. Inflammation and congestion ensues, with production of the characteristic white, fibrinous exudate. This discharge is the way the body relieves congestion and both recent and long-term lymphatic 'back log'.

Mind

If a person is 'recycling rubbish' at a physical level, it reflects a recycling of 'old stuff' at an emotional and mental level. These old mental and emotional patterns and beliefs are outdated but unfortunately stick around and are as difficult to release as the tenacious mucus that is their ultimate physical manifestation and final means of expression. Thank God for phlegm!!

Head

White, powdery dandruff often responds well to Kali Mur over a period of time. So does headache when there is associated nausea resulting from the presence of white milk-like mucus in the gut which may be vomited up during the headache. For any 'sick' or bilious headache resulting from overindulgence, Kali Mur should be considered after or with Nat Sulph.

Eyes, ears, and upper respiratory tract

The presence of a thick white mucous discharge in any of these areas* is always indicative of the need for Kali Mur. Chronic catarrh of the middle ear* when quality of hearing is affected because of swelling, congestion and closure is another indication. Kali Mur has a selective action on the middle ear, especially catarrh of the Eustachian tube which is often accompanied by crackling noises on blowing one's nose or swallowing. The presence of enlarged lymph glands of the neck, swollen adenoids and/or chronically enlarged tonsils* especially with associated white pustules all suggest Kali Mur.

Ulcers with a white-greyish, pustular centre are also an indication.

Tongue

A generally greyish-WHITE (often slimy) coated tongue is an indicator for Kali Mur, especially when associated with thrush of the mouth.

Gut

If digestive problems are present, Kali Mur can help recondition organs and glands associated with the digestive process. It is best taken with other tissue salts, e.g. Nat Phos, Nat Sulph, Mag Phos, depending on specific digestive symptoms.

Respiratory system

When a respiratory illness has advanced to the second stage* and there is production of thick, tenacious white phlegm, then Kali Mur should be employed. Associated with it may be wheezing and rattling which are characteristic signs of mucous congestion.

Female

Any congestion in the pelvic area creating a very dark, clotted and excessive menstrual flow, or a thick, milky-white bland discharge (leucorrhoea)* is a strong indication of need for the decongestive properties of Kali Mur.

Male

For soft, spongy enlargement of the prostate gland* consider Kali Mur. NB: Silica and/or Calc Fluor should be considered when the enlargement is indurated (hard).*

Urinary system

Chronic recurring cystitis* and the consistent presence of a thick, white mucus associated with the second stage of inflammation requires Kali Mur.

Structural system

Chronic swelling of joints* causing pain, especially rheumatic pain at night when slowing down and attempting to rest are indications for Kali Mur among other tissue salts. The heat of the bed may be found to aggravate these rheumatic pains.

Tissues

Kali Mur is the chief tissue salt for any soft glandular swelling.* (Calc Fluor and Silica for hard swellings.) For swelling of tissues resulting from injury Kali Mur is indicated with or after Ferrum Phos. Also consider Kali Mur for ill effects of vaccination* such as the presence of warts, and especially for long-term immunological effects such as lymphatic congestion.

Always remember that a sticky, white or sometimes white-greyish discharge exuding from any body tissue* is the prime indication for Kali Mur.

Skin

The skin is an organ in itself, and skin problems therefore indicate a need for the organ reconditioner, Kali Mur. Acne, abscesses, boils, vesicular eruptions and eczema, especially when there is swelling and the characteristic thick, white discharge are all good indications for the use of Kali Mur. Additional tissue salts will always be needed for skin problems, depending on individual symptoms related to colour of discharge, sensations, and aggravating or ameliorating factors.

General
Worse by:

Rheumatic ailments that respond to Kali Mur are often worse on initial movement and at night. Fatty, rich food is not tolerated if there is a congested liver involvement.

Complementary and related salts

Kali Mur complements Ferrum Phos for immune dysfunction and ongoing inflammatory states.

Ferrum Phos is recognised as the tissue salt for first stage disease or infection, Kali Mur for second stage, and Kali Sulph for third stage. It should be noted that these stages of disease can exist concurrently in the body.

Supportive measures

A change of environment, for example in the form of a holiday or different work can help to shift old, stagnant patterns.

Gentle aerobic exercise and walking at an unhurried pace will help balance body-mind activity and facilitate lymphatic (waste) movement and processing. Massage would have the same effect.

Work, rest (especially mental) and play need to be in good balance, and sufficient sleep is essential. Slow down and see how it feels!

Diet

Good sources of potassium chloride are asparagus, green beans, silver beet, carrots, cauliflower, celery, sweet corn, peaches, apricots, pineapples, plums. Herbs to consider are phytolacca, yarrow and violet.

Flower essences

Cerato (Bach) helps reduce self-doubt in order to get in touch with your own truths, living and following a path in life that is truly of your own design. It helps release old 'congested' patterns that no longer serve a new more assured purpose. Red Clover (FES) also helps release old, obsolete patterns of thinking and feeling, especially those related to fears associated with past trauma. White Chestnut (Bach) for persistent worry, and Star of Bethlehem (Bach) for old, unresolved shock, can be thought of for the same reasons. Boronia (Aus Bush) could be considered to help release old, obsessive thoughts.

Related disciplines

Iridology

A classical indication in the iris for Kali Mur is the presence of a lymphatic 'rosary', i.e. signs of lymphatic congestion. Any other sign of organ congestion will also warrant the use of Kali Mur.

Astrology

Kali Mur assists Gemini people whose vitality is more on the mental level than the physical. Quick actions, constant alertness and rapidly changing thoughts can lead to a scattering of nervous energy. This overstimulation, and often lack of connection with and care of the body, creates opportunities for Kali Mur related illnesses to arise. If Uranian activity dominates in any individual the same problems can easily develop.

Keywords

Glandular tonic, congestion remover, blood and lymphatic conditioner; facilitates and resolves second stage of inflammation.

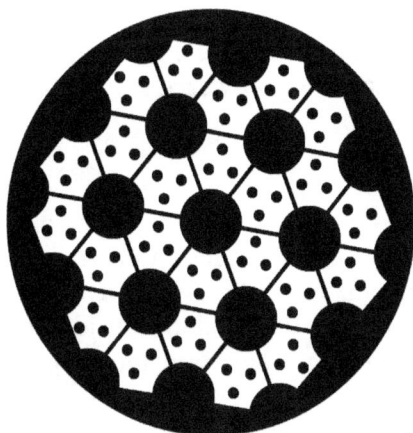

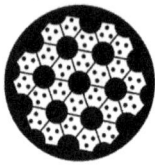

Kali Phos

Potassium phosphate

Potassium phosphate is a constituent of all body fluids and is essential for the formation and proper maintenance of tissue. It has a notable action in the brain (especially the grey matter), nerves, muscle and blood cells. The tissue salt is the great nerve nutrient and tonic.

It also has an antiseptic action and hinders decay of tissues especially as a result of deficient innervation in the areas resulting from lack of activity, paralysis or immobilisation of limbs.

Body type

Long-term deficiency of potassium phosphate may present in someone who is tired, weak and exhausted but at the same time hypersensitive and on edge. The person may say that they have always suffered from 'nerves', manifesting in symptoms such as insomnia, bouts of depression, nervous headaches and pains and nervous exhaustion. All these symptoms call for Kali Phos, and the remedy will be equally useful even when they are not part of a long-term picture.

Another common use for Kali Phos is during convalescence, especially when the thought of going back to work seems overwhelming.

Mind

Of the twelve tissue salts, Kali Phos is the prime remedy to consider for mentally related symptoms.* In particular, it may be useful in cases of anticipatory anxiety and nervous dread that seem to have no special cause. Kali Phos is the tissue salt to consider for overstimulated and irritated states of mind and depressed and pessimistic states that may follow.

Brain fag in mentally overtaxed students and loss of memory in general are indications for the use of Kali Phos. Always consider it, with Mag Phos, for nervous tension, insomnia, especially from over-tiredness, and burn-out after prolonged stress. Those needing Kali Phos often display a kind of shyness because they are too tired to respond socially. These people desire company of an undemanding nature – maybe just someone in the next room!

Head and face

Cerebral fatigue related to potassium imbalance can lead to vertigo and headache accompanied by confusion, inability to think, irritability and exhaustion. Nervous headache from loss of sleep or excessive mental work is an indication for Kali Phos. So is headache with an empty 'all gone' feeling in the stomach.

Consider Kali Phos with Mag Phos for neuralgic pains,* or on its own when Mag Phos fails.

Eyes

Some Kali Phos indications are weak eyesight from mental exhaustion and drooping eyelids from lack of muscle tone due to weakness of nerves in the area. (Think of Calc Fluor when this symptom is due to a general lack of tissue tone).

NB: Any disturbance or perversion of senses* through overstimulation or nervous exhaustion strongly suggests Kali Phos.

Gut

One characteristic of the need for Kali Phos can be excessive hunger even after eating: the nervous 'all gone' feeling in the stomach remains. All types of nervous sensation located in the stomach, e.g. feelings of 'butterflies in the stomach' before an important event, can be indications for the use of Kali Phos. Indigestion and flatulence after eating while in a state of nervous tension often respond well. Also consider Mag Phos.

Respiratory system

Kali Phos is an extremely important tissue salt in long-term treatment of nervous asthma.* With Mag Phos, it helps firstly to normalise an overstimulated nervous system resulting in asthmatic spasm and shortness of breath, and secondly to strengthen and tone the depressed nervous system associated with chronic asthma.*

Circulatory system

Kali Phos can be considered for cerebral circulatory insufficiency resulting in faintness and dizziness in nervous people.* Also consider Kali Phos with Mag Phos and perhaps others for palpitation that arises from exertion and emotional causes.*

Female

For painful menses* with associated depression, lassitude, and nervous debility always consider Kali Phos along with Mag Phos.

Male

Impotence* after prolonged mental stress, increased sexual desire with reduced potency, and severe prostration after sexual excess are all conditions calling for Kali Phos.

Urinary system

Consider Kali Phos if Calc Phos alone fails to assist cases of enuresis in nervous children.

Structural system

Use Kali Phos for any type of paralysis* or sensations of numbness or lameness in any part of the body,* especially if there is some improvement with gentle motion. After traumatic damage to any highly innervated part of the body, e.g. fingers or spine,* Kali Phos will assist the recovery of the damaged nerve tissue.

Tissues

Kali Phos is the primary tissue salt for cases of atrophy of limbs from lack of use or disease. When septic conditions develop,* consider Kali Phos with Calc Phos. Remember Kali Phos acts as an antiseptic, so always consider it whenever putrid or foul discharges* are present.

Skin

Stress-related alopecia* is often helped by Kali Phos. In fact all skin irritations and complaints directly related to stress or nervous states should respond to this tissue salt, usually in conjunction with others.

Sleep

For sleeplessness from worry, nervous anticipation, overstimulation, night terrors, irritability or any emotional upset consider Kali Phos. Think of it also for somnambulism after long illness or nervous exhaustion. In children, symptoms such as sleepwalking and nightmares may be accompanied by bed-wetting in some cases.

General
Better by:
All conditions requiring Kali Phos are temporarily relieved by rest and nourishment. Mindfulness and relaxation techniques also help, as does gentle motion such as walking, and pleasant, undemanding company.

Worse by:
Excitement (including excessive sexual activity), worry, mental and physical exertion, COLD, especially cold air and noise tend to aggravate Kali Phos conditions.

Complementary and related salts
Mag Phos complements Kai Phos for nervous problems.

Kali Phos is related to Calc Fluor in its ability to 'tone' body and mind. Calc Fluor is used when decrease in tone is due to lack of elasticity or slackness in tissue structure. Kali Phos assists when lack of tone is due to deficient innervation of tissues.

Supportive measures
Rest (especially mental rest), fresh air, and gentle physical exercise, preferably, out of doors, e.g. easy WALKING with no particular destination.

Nourish your body as well as your mind.

The colour red in all forms may be used to stimulate a depleted nervous system.

Meditation may help you hear the relaxing tune in your heart rather than the disturbing racket in your head!

Diet
Good sources of potassium phosphate are lettuce, cauliflower, olives, spinach, onions, mustard, walnuts, lentils, radishes, horseradish, tomatoes, potatoes, lemons, apples and dates. Some herbs rich in potassium phosphate are gentian, hops, avena, garlic, ginger and St John's Wort.

Flower essences

Impatiens (Bach) can help those who are driven to nervous exhaustion in relentless pursuit of goals and deadlines. It can also assist relaxation, making it possible to relinquish an unrelenting sense of urgency.

In conditions requiring Kali Phos, Aloe Vera (FES) for 'burn-out', Lemon and Peppermint (both FES) to help 'tone up', Macrocarpa (Aus Bush) and Olive (Bach) for nervous exhaustion may help.

Related disciplines

Iridology

The iris of someone with a long-standing need of Kali Phos will most commonly display a dilated or 'ballooning' autonomic nerve wreath. What also often presents is a single deeply 'engraved' dark nerve ring, in contrast to the multiple nerve rings of Mag Phos which are usually lighter in colour. Combined characteristics of both these types of nerve ring may occur, indicating a need for both tissue salts.

Astrology

Aries mental and physical 'burn out' responds well to Kali Phos, as do the consequences of any abuse or overextension of fiery inner forces.

Keywords

Nerve nutrient, brain tonic; mentally calms and uplifts.

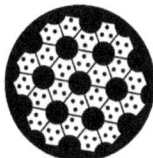

Kali Sulph

Potassium sulphate

Oxygen is taken up buy the iron in blood cells and is carried to every cell of the body by means of the action of potassium sulphate. Metabolic imbalances of this mineral create problems in the skin's epidermal cells, causing scaly eruptions that often have a humid, sticky base, and in the epithelial cells of mucous membranes, producing profuse, yellow and yellow-greenish, slightly irritating discharges.

It is the tissue salt for third stage infection or inflammation-regressive suppuration.* This is usually the stage at which antibiotics are administered in conventional medicine.

Mind

Those in need of Kali Sulph may present as irritable, hurried and easily angered. Somatisation of this temperament in the form of 'irritation' of skin or mucous membranes can often bring relief on the mental level. Congestion in the head, for example of the sinuses, may be accompanied by confusion and a thick, 'fuzzy' feeling preventing clear thinking.

Head

Headache of those needing Kali Sulph is often begun or made worse by a warm, stuffy atmosphere. Dandruff, scaly scalp and falling hair are all indications that skin integrity is compromised, making Kali Sulph an important component of treatment. Consider it also for poor hair quality indicating that the 'soil' (the skin) it is growing in is substandard.

Eyes

Visual disturbances* associated with sinus and sinus-related migraine can be a good indicator for Kali Sulph.

Ears

Think of Kali Sulph for chronic catarrhal deafness and/or earache* associated with periodic or persistent yellow discharge. (If the discharge contains pus or is blood-streaked think Calc Sulph.)

57

Upper respiratory tract

In late, consolidating stages of inflammation and infection* when a yellow or yellow-greenish discharge has developed, Kali Sulph is the prime tissue salt to consider. Yellow post-nasal drip, hawking up of yellow-green mucus, or nasal passages blocked with tenacious yellow-green discharge are all strong indications for Kali Sulph.

Tongue

A slimy, creamy-yellow coating over the tongue, especially at its rear, lends support for the prescription of Kali Sulph.

Gut

If Mag Phos fails to provide relief from sugar cravings or colic pain, Kali Sulph should be considered. Feelings of pressure, fullness and sometimes burning in the lower abdomen associated with bowel gas of a sulphurous odour are good reasons to consider Kali Sulph. Intense itching of the anus may also be present.

Respiratory system

Infections, inflammatory states and spasm (caused by anything from bronchitis to asthma*) accompanied by yellow-green expectoration warrant the use of Kali Sulph. There may be rattling mucus in the chest. Another characteristic symptom of the need for Kali Sulph is that conditions are worse in a warm atmosphere.

Urinary system

For chronic cystitis* where a yellowy discharge indicates that infection has reached the third stage, consider Kali Sulph.

Structural system

Use Kali Sulph to supplement the action of Mag Phos in cases of neuralgia* and rheumatism, especially if pains shift and wander.

Tissues

The characteristic expression of a need for Kali Sulph is a yellow, sticky, slimy excretion from either mucus membranes or skin.

Skin

Psoriasis* where skin is dry and scaly, or eczema* which burns and itches and has a yellow, or less frequently a watery exudate often responds well to Kali Sulph. Chronic tinea resulting in septic states* and sometimes malformations of toenails or fingernails is another indication for long-term treatment with Kali Sulph. Silica may also be considered.

General
Better by:
Kali Sulph conditions are always improved by fresh, cool air and by being outside. People in need of Kali Sulph crave to be outside and moving around.

Worse by:
HEATED ROOMS, air, or weather aggravate. Symptoms are usually worse in the evenings.

Complementary and related skills
Ferrum Phos and Kali Sulph can complement each other to improve the integrity of mucous membranes, especially those of the respiratory tract.

Kali Sulph and Calc Sulph conditions both have discharges but those of the latter are more pustular and may be blood-streaked.

Kali Sulph's action on the third stage of inflammation and infection relates to Ferrum Phos and Kali Mur, which are prescribed for the first and second stages respectively. Note that these stages can occur simultaneously in various parts of the body.

Supportive measures
Go back to basics and consider diet. As well as looking at food rich in potassium sulphate, try to 'liven up' sluggish digestion, perhaps with the addition of fermented foods to your diet. Most of all consider lifestyle and how it might be draining nervous energy. Remember, if you are having difficulty coping with and 'digesting' life, you will have difficulty digesting food.

Allow the 'inner child' out to play – even to misbehave – more often!

Diet

Very good sources of potassium sulphate are chicory, carrots, oats, rye, whole wheat, endive, lettuce, cheese and almonds. Herbs rich in potassium sulphate are PULSATILLA, hydrastis (golden seal) and licorice.

Flower essences

White Chestnut (Bach) has often proved useful for the cluttered, thought-congested mind that can accompany catarrhal congestion of the head. Centaury (Bach) and Larkspur (FES) both help to change old, reactionary patterns and 'knee-jerk' responses. New, more vital responses to people and life in general can then allow the body to follow suit, responding in more effective ways to infection and the accumulation of toxins.

Related disciplines

Iridology

A dark, under-active scurf rim may indicate the need for Kali Sulph. Also any indication or the presence of chronic infection, e.g. yellowy-brown areas in the iris, is a sign that it might be useful to consider Kali Sulph.

Astrology

Sensitive areas of Virgo constitutions are mucous membranes of the small intestine (bowel), parts of the gut that produce digestive enzymes, and the liver. Health in these areas can suffer as a result of worry, anxiety and environmental influences which deplete the nervous system and reduce recuperative capacity, leaving the body vulnerable to infection and prolonged inflammatory states.

Keywords

Cell oxygenator (with Ferrum Phos); membrane normaliser and conditioner.

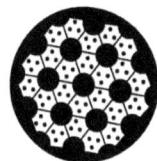

Nat Mur

Sodium chloride

Sodium chloride is a constituent of every liquid and solid in the body. It regulates moisture content of cells by virtue of its role as water distributor. It maintains the body's water balance by regulating osmosis – the movement of fluids in and out of cells.

Body type

The 'retentive' nature of those in need of Nat Mur is evident at all levels. However, those whose symptoms are on mental and emotional planes are likely to respond better to higher homeopathic potencies. Those who are sensitive to lower homeopathic potencies of this mineral in tissue salt form are more likely to be prone to physical symptoms such as fluid retention in one part of the body and dryness in another.

People needing Nat Mur are often thin, especially in the upper part of the body, despite a very good appetite and sometimes intense thirst.

Mind

People who require Nat Mur can become sad, depressed and pessimistic, especially when they are run-down and tired. They may prefer to be left alone to think through their problems; consolation only makes them more moody, with a stronger preference for being alone. For best results, prescribe Nat Mur when there are physical symptoms to support your diagnosis. If these are absent, Nat Mur in tissue salt form may not be as effective for mental symptoms alone as higher homeopathic potencies.

Head

Nat Mur is the chief tissue salt remedy for sunstroke.*In this condition, heat of the sun causes dehydration and fluid imbalance in the affected area calling for Nat Mur. The characteristic headache of Nat Mur is present on waking after a night of unrefreshing sleep, and reaches its peak by mid-morning. There may be constipation with a dry crumbly stool – more evidence of fluid imbalance, in this case limiting water content which assists easy passing of stools.

Eyes

Any affection causing production of a profuse clear, watery mucus or flow of tears from the eyes* warrants consideration of Nat Mur.

Ears

There may be deafness from internal swelling* that has usually arisen suddenly, e.g. from an allergic reaction. Ferrum Phos and Kali Mur should also be considered.

Upper respiratory tract

Nasal catarrh with significant loss of sense of smell and taste is an indication for Nat Mur (also Kali Phos). Catarrh associated with common cold; salty, free flowing and watery or like raw egg white, or mucous catarrh produced in abnormal quantities – copiousness being the significant factor – are strong indications for prescribing Nat Mur. Frequent sneezing associated with free-flowing, watery secretions, e.g. hay fever, often responds well.

Tongue

'Mapped' tongue may indicate a need for either Nat Mur or Calc Fluor depending on other symptoms.

Gut

An imbalance of sodium chloride in the system may result in craving for or strong aversion to salt. Nat Mur can correct problems arising from excessive intake of table salt such as excessive thirst (or hunger) or no thirst at all. Craving for or strong aversion to bread may be present. Excessive salivation or a watery, non-acidic reflux from the stomach may be an indication for Nat Mur, as is excessive fluid production anywhere in the body.*

At the other extreme, when the lips (especially the lower lip) and corners of the mouth are dry and cracked, Nat Mur often helps. It is the prime tissue salt used for the treatment of cold sores. Best results are achieved when the remedy is taken over a number of months.

Respiratory system

Production of copious, clear, frothy, and watery phlegm, often loose and rattling,* gives a good indication for the use of Nat Mur, usually in conjunction with other tissue salts.

Circulatory system

Cold extremities can be a feature of constitutions with a long-standing need for Nat Mur. So is a strong sensitivity to and dislike for extremes of temperature – hot or cold.

Female

Consider Nat Mur for irregular and missed periods,* especially when associated with emotional upset or over-excitement in pubescent girls or young women. It is also useful in cases of scanty periods when associated with other Nat Mur-related symptoms.

Urinary system

When there is persistent excessive production of watery urine,* consider Nat Mur.

Tissues

Watery exudations in excessive amounts* are key indications for the use of Nat Mur. Emaciation, especially of tissues of the upper body can occur, even while living and eating well.

Skin

Nat Mur has been used effectively for all affections producing watery vesicles that are often small and blister like, and for thin whitish scaling of the skin. Also consider Nat Mur for skin that takes on an oily appearance, particularly in the face and forehead, but is excessively dry in other areas. Herpetic eruptions, shingles*(use with Mag Phos), and the effects of insect bites have all responded well to Nat Mur.

General

Better by:

Those who need Nat Mur much prefer the open air and being outside. They nearly always feel better being alone.

Worse by:

Symptoms and indeed general well-being are often worse in the morning, especially before 10 a.m.

They are also worse at the seaside (salty atmosphere), worse with heat despite being cold-sensitive, worse when someone attempts to console, and prone to cyclic aggravations. Mental work can often bring on headaches.

Complementary and related salts

Nat Mur is related in its action, and often complements Ferrum Phos in initial stages of inflammation when the discharge is clear and free-flowing, e.g. the start of a head cold.

Supportive measures

Aerobic exercise is useful to stimulate circulation at ALL levels of being. Relaxation techniques involving breathing exercises can be helpful for the same reason, and also because they encourage release and the ability to 'let go'.

Avoid the addition of crude salt (sodium chloride) to food and drink.

Forgive but don't forget.

Diet

Good sources of sodium chloride are seafoods (although some people requiring Nat Mur develop allergies and intolerances to them), cabbage, celery, carrots, figs, apples, spinach, asparagus, strawberries, lentils, meat, almonds and sesame seeds (tahini).

Herbs rich in a useful form of sodium chloride are marigold, witch hazel, comfrey, mistletoe and valerian.

Flower essences

For habits of emotional retention consider Willow (Bach) to help release old hurts and grievances. Water Violet (Bach) can help those who have become emotionally aloof and self-contained to preserve their 'watery' emotional and sensitive nature.

Related disciplines

Iridology

A 'sodium' ring in the outer part of the iris is the clearest indication for Nat Mur (but always consider the other sodium salts as well: Nat Phos and Nat Sulph), reflecting an accumulation of salt in tissues and blood vessels, either from excessive salt intake in diet, or problems with proper metabolism of salt. Nat Mur will help correct both excess and imbalance.

Astrology

Nat Mur is the tissue salt for Aquarians; on a physical level in relation to flow and distribution of water in the body, and on a metaphysical level relating to the flow of etheric energies through the subtle body. A sodium chloride imbalance invariably results in some kind of circulatory problem.

Keywords

Water distribution and balance.

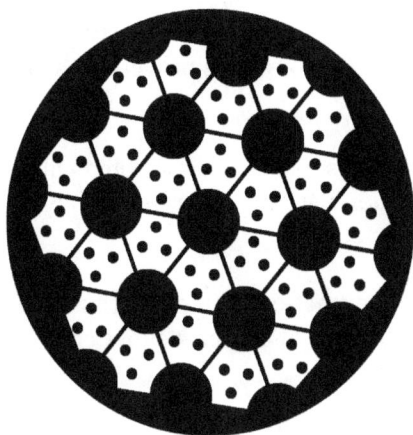

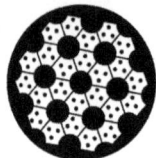

Nat Phos

Sodium phosphate

Sodium phosphate is present in blood, muscles, nerves and brain cells, and in the fluid between cells. It splits lactic acid into carbonic acid and water, reducing acid in the system. All physical complaints relating to hyper-acidity will respond to Nat Phos. It also has a particular effect on regulation of bile consistency.

Body type

The classical picture of an ongoing imbalance in sodium phosphate is that of someone who suffers from over-acidity. This may take the form of anything from recurring heartburn to chronic inflammatory states of rheumatic nature. An over-acidic system creates a tendency to inflammatory conditions and inhibits their resolution.

Mind

Acidity at a physical level can reflect suppression of fiery energies on a more subtle level. Frustration results when these energies are unable to find a creative outlet, and this may manifest in occasional outbursts of misplaced anger or as the proverbial 'acid' tongue.

Head

Whenever there is headache associated with vomiting and gastric problems consider Nat Phos together with Nat Sulph.

Eyes

Nat Phos in conjunction with other tissue salts has often proved helpful for discharges of golden-yellow, creamy matter from the eyes*

Upper respiratory tract

A yellow, creamy, acid discharge from the nose causing itching and irritation often responds well to the use of Nat Phos.

Tongue

A creamy or golden-yellow coating at the back of the tongue is a clear indication of a need for Nat Phos.

Teeth

Children or adults who grind their teeth in sleep are often indicating an over-acid system and therefore a need for Nat Phos. They are agitated by something(s) 'grinding' away at the psyche – things that may find no avenue of expression during waking hours.

Gut

Any form of hyper-acidity including sour reflux (or vomiting) from the stomach, dyspepsia, heartburn and acid eructations are certain indications for the use of Nat Phos. Other important indications are nausea and vomiting of sour foods (also Nat Sulph), sour, burning stools in cases of diarrhoea, and virtually any digestive complaint.

Female

Vaginal secretions* of an acidic nature that create irritation and redness, or that are creamy, yellow and sour-smelling suggest Nat Phos as a natural choice.

Urinary system

Burning urination* reflects overly acid urine and hence Nat Phos is strongly indicated. If there is a diagnosis of cystitis, Ferrum Phos would be prescribed to address the inflammatory condition.

Structural system

Consider Nat Phos for rheumatic and arthritic problems resulting from an acid build-up in the body, especially gout* and the like. Remember an overly acid system makes one more prone to inflammatory conditions and encourages crystalline deposits to form on bones and joints, causing cracking of the joints.

Tissues

Nat Phos is generally an excellent remedy for liver and digestive conditions.

Consider it for any sign of jaundice* characterised by yellowness of the skin and tissues.

Skin

Yellowing of the skin; hives, especially after eating acid foods such as oranges; dryness of skin; and episodes of skin 'itching all over' can be indications for the use of Nat Phos. When secretions are yellow and honey-like you would do well to consider Nat Phos among other well chosen tissue salts.

General

Worse by:

Changeable weather can be uncomfortable for those with a sodium phosphate imbalance, especially for rheumatic complaints. When there is a sluggish liver, fatty, rich and acid-producing foods including sugar, alcohol and excess heavy protein such as that found in meat and dairy products are generally not well-tolerated. Open air is preferred to calm weather.

Complementary and related salts

Nat Phos and Nat Sulph combine well for most digestive disturbances.

Nat Phos will enhance assimilation of any other tissue salt when the system is excessively acid.

Mag Phos and Calc Phos can play an important role along with Nat Phos in maintaining a proper acid-alkaline balance in the body.

Supportive measures

Learn about acid-alkaline balance in diet, and learn about alkaline foods.

Gentle aerobic and breath balancing exercise are important. Explore creative outlets where you feel free and safe to go with 'gut' feelings and respond uninhibitedly to your inner senses.

Don't worry about it yet – it might not happen!

Diet

Good sources of sodium phosphate are apples, figs, carrots, celery, asparagus, white rice, silver beet, corn, berries, almonds and resins.

Herbs rich in sodium phosphate are alfalfa, violet, lemon balm, the mints and pennyroyal.

Flower essences

Scleranthus (Bach) is a great balancer of thoughts and emotions and this can have a balancing effect on the physical level. It can help a person to externalise frustrated fiery energy in a decisive and creative way. Fear of taking action or making decisions because of potential consequences or effects on others can be inhibiting. Mimulus (Bach), Tansy and Dill (both FES) may assist in taking decisive actions to deal with frustrations, and so can Red Grevillia (Aust Bush).

Related disciplines

Iridology

For any 'acid' signs, usually depicted by white flaring of the iris, Nat Phos is strongly indicated. Also if the gut area displays toxicity or poor assimilation consider Nat Phos with other tissue salts – tongue presentation will give guidance here.

Astrology

Libran energy is symbolised by the scales of balance and when out of balance, Librans are given to fear, worry and indecision. The acid condition in the body tends to increase, making them vulnerable to problems associated with hyper-acidity. Too much thinking, worrying and weighing up options is characteristic of excess of the air element, 'fanning' the fire (element) that begins to burn out of control deep within the psyche.

Keywords

Acid neutraliser; acid-alkaline balancer.

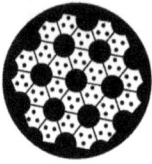

Nat Sulph

Sodium sulphate

While sodium chloride redistributes water for most effective use in the organism, sodium sulphate eliminates excessive water in tissues, blood and other body fluids. It has been called nature's water purifier, because although it is not present in the cells themselves, only in intercellular fluid, it acts as their 'environmental cleanser', helping remove pollutants and so assisting the liver in its role as detoxifier – a mammoth task in this day and age.

It also stimulates epithelial cells in the bile duct, pancreas and intestinal canal, facilitating normal levels of secretion in these important digestive organs. Over-production or under-production of secretions may develop when there is an imbalance of sodium sulphate.

The characteristic discharge is either yellowish and watery or greenish and thick but is nearly always irritating.

Deficiency or imbalance of sodium sulphate also affects epithelial cells of respiratory mucous membranes. Nat Sulph is prescribed as a preventative in chronic respiratory ailments.*

Body type

Those with a long-standing need for Nat Sulph may tend towards obesity, especially of the abdomen, thighs and buttocks. These areas in particular are prone to becoming oedematous, i.e. tissues become infiltrated by water and lipids (fats) creating cellulite.

'Congestive' liver symptoms are common, and over time rheumatic ailments tend to develop.

All problems are aggravated by exposure to humidity.

Mind

Nat Sulph has 'retention' tendencies on all levels, perhaps to an even greater degree than Nat Mur, the other tissue salt sharing this symptom-picture. Sadness, depression and sometimes loathing of life as a consequence of holding on to old hurts are states of mind that are all too familiar. As with Nat Mur, physical symptoms must also be present for appropriate prescription. Depressive moods are often worse from emotion-provoking atmospheres created by such things as music. This susceptibility translates onto the physical level as extreme sensitivity to moisture or damp atmospheres – water being the element that symbolises emotion – most pronounced in rheumatic conditions.

Head

Ailments that arise after head or spinal injuries* whether of recent or remote origin, especially persistent headaches or symptoms of a mental nature, e.g. increased forgetfulness, may be helped by taking Nat Sulph over an extended period. Immediate and frequent administration of Nat Sulph is indicated in headaches associated with biliousness, nausea and vomiting of bile, and/or colic pains and diarrhoea.*

Upper respiratory tract

For any thick, yellow or salty (think also Nat Mur) mucous discharge consider Nat Sulph if other symptoms support this choice.

Tongue

A dirty yellowish-brown or yellowish-grey coating is the most characteristic tongue sign for Nat Sulph. However a clear and clean-looking tongue may also present in the 'fluid-filled' or oedematous person.

Gut

Some key symptoms that would strongly indicate the usefulness of Nat Sulph are a bitter taste in the mouth and biliousness from excess bile production leading to vomiting of greenish, bitter fluids. Other key symptoms are flatulent colic with pronounced abdominal bloating and intolerance of tight clothing around the abdomen. Intense thirst for cold drinks may also be present.

The liver may be engorged, sensitive and sore to touch,* especially when lying on the left side.

Watery, diarrhoea-like stools, associated with much wind, and especially urgent in the early morning are good indications for Nat Sulph. Sometimes there may be alternating diarrhoea and constipation with large, hard stools.

Respiratory system

Bronchitis or asthma* that is notably worse when there is a change to damp weather or humid conditions suggests the use of Nat Sulph. Thick, greenish expectoration is characteristic. Best results are achieved by using higher homeopathic potencies as a preventative measure, under the guidance of a fully qualified homeopath.

Nat Sulph in conjunction with Kali Mur and other tissue salts often helps reduce discomfort of aching limbs associated with influenza.

Structural system

For rheumatic pains in joints, especially the lower back, hips, knees and ankles, aggravated by damp and humid conditions, always consider Nat Sulph. Pains are often helped by slow, progressively more vigorous movement.

As mentioned previously, consider the use of Nat Sulph for persons with functional problems after trauma to the head or spinal column.* (See 'Head')

Tissues

Oedematous states* are common in those with a sodium sulphate imbalance. Fluid retention is particularly prevalent in the feet.

General

Better by:

Those needing Nat Sulph feel much better in themselves in dry weather, and so do their symptoms. Rheumatic pains are reduced by changing position frequently.

Worse by:

Any exposure to DAMP or humid conditions – rain, proximity to water, at the seaside, warm humid winds, etc. – will cause aggravation. Tight abdominal clothing, especially when associated with overeating, will cause great discomfort.

Complementary and related salts

Nat Phos complements the action of Nat Sulph in most digestive, over-acidic and liver related problems.

Nat Mur and Nat Sulph are related: both have an important role in the body's water metabolism.

Both Kali Mur and Nat Sulph are important for the proper function of organs and glands.

Supportive measures

Anything that encourages breaking up of physical and emotional congestion will assist those in need of Nat Sulph. NATURAL stimulants such as physical exercise, light-hearted, humorous company and entertainment and a colourful environment are some ways to get life-energies flowing.

Cleansing diets will be useful, but remember to stay light-hearted and creative when developing your healthy diet and lifestyle.

Don't play the same old record all the time!

Diet

Rich sources of sodium sulphate are found in silver beet, spinach, cabbage, cauliflower, onion, pumpkin, horseradish, cucumber, celery and apple. Herbs rich in sodium sulphate are yarrow, berberis, lycopodium and burdock.

Flower essences

Those in need of Nat Sulph may suffer from a sluggish metabolism which makes them prone to putting on weight and becoming generally discouraged. Over-indulgence, especially in rich foods, encourages this tendency. Gentian (Bach) may help those who are discouraged and depressed for these reasons. Tansy (FES) can help develop a more enduringly motivated attitude to personal health and well-being in those who tend to procrastinate and feel 'stuck'. Cayenne (FES) and Old Man Banksia (Aus Bush) may also act as catalysts for those struggling to take positive measures towards achieving a better and more healthy lifestyle.

Related disciplines

Iridology

A toxic expression in the area of the iris associated with gut symptoms, and congestive liver signs are usually a good indication for Nat Sulph. Consider this tissue salt if there are signs of glandular congestion anywhere, especially in the skin area.

Astrology

Taurian natures can often be helped by Nat Sulph to modify problems outlined in the section on flower essences. It can act, for Taureans, as a regulator of body fluids, and as a helpful liver detoxifier.

Keywords

Eliminates excess water; 'environmental cleanser' of cells, liver decongestant.

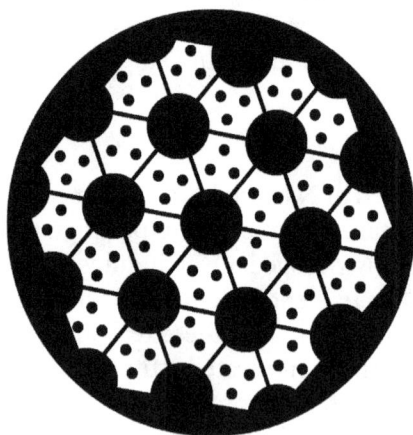

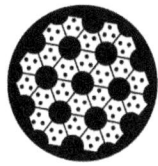

Guide to symptomatic prescribing

The first choice of tissue salt(s) for symptoms is written in **Bold**. Other tissue salts to consider as well as, as an alternative to or when the first choice is unsuccessful are written in *italic*.

Nervous system including mental symptoms

Anxiety*: **KP**
• in children: **CP**, *KP*
• Addiction*: **MP, KP**
Brain Fag: **KP**, *S*
Brooding: **KP**, *NS, NM*
Concentration poor:
• in children: **CP, MP**, *KP, S*
• in adults: **KP, MP**
Cramps: **MP, CP**
Difficult to think*: **KP**, *S*
Dizziness*: **FP**, *KP*
Depression*, Despondency: **KP**
Distorted sensory perception*: **KP**, *MP, S*
Fainting*, nervous reaction: **KP**, *FP, S*
Fright, effects from: **KP**
Globus Hystericus*, nervous reaction: **KP**, *MP*
Hiccough: **MP**
Hypersensitivity*: **MP, KP**, *S*
• to light: **MP**, *KP*
• to noise: **S**, *KP*
• to pain: **KP, MP**, *CP, S*
Hysteria*: **KP, MP**, *NM*
Home-sickness: **KP**, *NM*

Irritability
• in children: **CP, MP**, *FP*
• in adults: **KP, MP**, *FP, CP*
Melancholic mood swings*:
NM, *NS, KP*
Memory poor*: **KP**, *CP, MP, FP*
Mental symptoms predominate*: **KP**
Involuntary motion of limbs*: **MP**
Nervousness: **KP, MP**, *S*
Nerve damage*: **KP, MP, FP**, *CP, S*
Neuralgia*: **MP, KP, S, FP**, *NM*
• with inflammation: **FP**
• better with heat: **MP**
• not better with heat or cold: **S**
• shifting pains: **KS**
• with depression or weakness: **KP**
• periodic: **NM, MP**
Night terrors*: **KP**
Oversensitive: **MP, KP**, *S*
Pain*: **MP, KP, CP, FP**, *S*
Paralysis*: **KP**
Sciatica*: **MP, KP**, *FP*
Shaking (Trembling etc.): **MP**
Shyness, extreme: **KP**
Sighing: **KP, NM**
Sleeplessness*: **MP**, *KP*
• after excitement: **FP, MP**, *KP*
• from worry: **KP**, *MP, FP*
• in children: **CP, MP**

Sleepwalking*: **KP**, *S*
Somnambulism*: **KP**
Spasmodic twitching: **MP**, *CP*
Stammering*: **MP**
Talking in sleep: **KP**, *S*
Twitching: **MP**
Weep easily: **KP, NM**

Head symptoms

Cold sensations over: **CP**
Dandruff: **KS**, *NM*
Dizziness*: **FP**, *KP*
Hair falling out*: **KP**, *S, NM*
• with stress: **KP**
Headache*:
• with biliousness or nausea: **NS**
• with confusion: **KP**
• with dry constipation: **NM**
• with heat or throbbing: **FP**
• with irritability: **KP, MP**
• with prostration: **KP**
• with sharp, shooting pains: **MP**
• with spasmodic pain: **MP**
• with tension: **MP**
• with weariness: **KP**
• *worse by:*
  heated or stuffy rooms: **KS**
  light, bright: **MP**, *KP*
  loss of sleep: **KP**
  mental work: **KP**
  puberty: **CP**, *NM*
• *better by:*
  pleasant company: **KP**
  cold applications: **FP**
  cool, open air: **KS**
  warm application: **MP**
  gentle motion: **KP**
Sensitive, sore scalp: **FP, MP**
Sunstroke*: **NM**
Sweat, excess*: **NM**, *CP, MP*
• children esp. at night: **CP**
• or lack of: **S**

Eye symptoms

Bloodshot: **FP**, *NP*
Blurred vision*:
• from eyestrain: **CF**
• from tension: **MP**
Burning*: **FP**
Cataracts*(overgrowth): **CF, S**
Discharge*:
• clear, fluent and tear-like: **NM**, *FP*
• white, thick: **KM**
• creamy-yellow, fluent: **NP**
• yellow, or yellow-green,
• thick and sticky: **KS**
• yellow, persistent, fluent (often blood streaked): **CS**
• yellow-green, recurring: **S**
Eyelids drooping*: **KP**, *CF*
Intolerance of bright light*: **MP**, *FP*
Inflammation*: **FP**, *KM*
• no discharge: **FP**
• discharge: refer above
Light sensitive*: **MP**
Pressure* (e.g. glaucoma): **KM**, *MP*
Pupils*:
• contracted: **MP**
• dilated: **KP**, *CF*
Styes: **S**
Tears in excess*:
• acrid: **NP**
• bland: **NM**
Twitching: **MP**, *CP*
Visual spots, sparks, flecks etc. before the eyes*: **MP**, *NS*

Ear symptoms

Burning in*: **NP**, *FP*, *KM*
Catarrh of ear*:
• causing deafness: **KS**
• of Eustachian tubes: **KS**
• of middle ear: **KM**, *FP*
Crackling noises on blowing nose or swallowing: **KM**
Deafness*:
• from congestion: **KM**
• from inflammation: **FP**, *KM*
• nervous: **KP**, *MP*
Discharge*:
• clear, watery: **NM**, *FP*
• albuminous (like egg white): **CP**, *FP*, *KM*
• grey or thick white: **KM**
• thick, yellow, bloody: **CS**
• foul, fetid, offensive: **KP**
Earache*: **FP**, *KM*
• with redness, heat and inflammation: **FP**
• with throbbing pain: **FP**
• with sharp shooting pain: **MP**, *FP*
• with discharge: refer above
• associated with swollen glands of neck and ear: **KM**, *FP*
Hearing difficulty*:
• with nervous exhaustion: **KP**
• with discharge: refer above
• from inflammation: **FP**

Nasal symptoms

Bleeding*: **FP**
• in weaker nervous constitutions: **KP**
Blood nose*: **FP**
Catarrh
• worse in warm or stuffy room: **KS**
• evening: **KS**
• post nasal drip: refer discharge (below)

Catches cold easily*: **FP**, *KM*
• in children: **FP**, **KM**, **CP**
Discharge*:
clear, watery (sometimes salty), fluent: **NM**
thick, albuminous discharge: **CP**
thick, white, not clear: **KM**
slimy yellow-greenish: **KS**
persistent, thick, yellow and blood-streaked: **CS**
fetid: **KP**
chronic, yellowish and fetid: **S**
Dryness and burning of nasal passages: **NS**, **FP**
First (inflammatory) stage of colds: **FP**
Loss of, or perversion of smell without catarrh*: **MP**, **KP**
Polyps*: **CP**, **KM**
Sneezing, frequently: **NM**

Mouth symptoms

Bad breath: **NS**, **NP**
Cracked lips*:
• with dryness: **NM**
• with a chronic tendency: **CF**
Glands swollen under tongue*: **KM**, **NM**
Gums*:
• bleed easily: **KP**, *FP*
• pale: **CP**
Gum-boil*:
• pustular: **S**, *CS*
• before pus: **KM**
Gums swollen*:
• hot and inflamed: **FP**
• with glands swollen: **KM**
• bleed easily: **KP**, *FP*
• pale: **CP**
Saliva, excessive: **NM**, *KM*
Taste:
• acid: **NP**

- bitter: **NS**
- insipid, disgusting: **CS**
- loss of: **NM**
- metallic: **NP**
- putrid: **KP**
- salty: **NM**
- sour: **NP**, *KM*
- sweetish: **CP**, *SP*

Thirst, excessive*: **NM**

Thrush*: **KM**

- with inflammation: **FP, KM**

Ulcers*:

- white: **KM**
- white and inflamed with redness: **FP, KM**
- ashy grey: **KP**

Tongue symptoms

Blisters (watery): **NM**

Clean, red and inflamed: **FP**

Coating:
- clear, frothy and watery: **NM**
- greyish-white: **KM**
- creamy or golden-yellow at base: **NP**
- yellow and slimy: **KS**
- greenish-brown or –grey at base
- (bitter taste): **NS**
- stale, brownish, mustard-like, offensive: **KP**

Cracked appearance: **CF**

Hardening or indurations*: **CF, S**

Inflammation, swelling:*: **FP**, *KM*
- with suppuration: **S, CS**

Numbness*: **CP**, *KP*

Ulcers: refer to '**Mouth**'

Vesicles (watery)*: **NM**

Dental symptoms

Ache*:
- with deep-seated pain: **S**, *MP*
- sharp, shooting pain: **MP**

- with swelling or inflammation: **KM, FP**
- worse from hot food/drink: **FP**
- worse with cold applications: **MP**
- better from hot applications: **MP**
- better from cold applications: **FP**

Decay tendency*: **CF**, *CP*

Detention retarded or problems associated*: **CP**

Enamel, brittle or deficient*: **CF**

Grinding*: **NP**, *MP*

Loose*: **CF**

Sensitive to cold or touch: **MP**, *CF*

Ulceration or abscess of roots*: **S**, *CS*

Throat symptoms

Adenoids*:
- chronic enlargement in children: **CP, KM, FP** (refer to tonsils also)

Burning*: **FP**

Constricted feeling (Globus Hystericus)*: **MP**

Hoarseness (from strain or overwork): **FP**, *CP*

Loss of voice*: **KM**

from strain: **FP**, *KM*

Red inflamed*: **FP**

Sore throat*:
- first stage (pain, heat, redness): **FP**
- with excessive dryness or watery secretion: **NM**
- associated with enlarged or tender glands: **KM**
- with swelling and grey-white patches: **KM**
- persistent suppuration: **CS**

Spasm*: **MP**

Tickling: **CP**, *CF*

Tonsils: (refer to sore throat also)
- recurring pustular formation: **S**
- chronic enlargement in children: **CP, FP, KM**

78

Ulceration*:
- with inflammation (red and sore): **FP**
- with white-grey discharge: **KM**

Stomach symptoms

Ache (pain)*:
- sore to touch: **CP**, *FP*
- with constipation: **KM**
- with loose bowls: **FP**, *CP*
- from eating even the smallest amount of food: **CP**
- with fever or inflammation: **FP**

Acidity: **NP**, *MP, CP*
- acid or sour reflux: **NP**

Appetite:
- lack of: **CP**
- never satisfied: **KP**

Belching: **MP, CP, NP**
- with sourness or bitterness: **NP**
- with regurgitation of food: **FP**

Bloated (with gas): **CP, NS**

Burning: **NP**, *CP, MP, FP*

Cold food/drink:
- relieves symptoms: **FP**
- aggravates symptoms: **MP, CP**

Colic or cramping*: **MP**, *CP*

Craving:
- for salty food/drink: **NM**
- for sweets: **MP**, *KS, S*
- for savoury things: **CP**

Distended (loosening clothes brings some relief): **NS**, *CP*

Fatty food disagrees: **KM**, *NP*

Heartburn*: **NP**, *FP, MP, CP, S*

Hiccough: **MP**

Hungry feeling after eating: **KP**

Migraine (children)*: **MP, CP**

Morning sickness*: **NP**
- with cravings: **MP**

Nausea*:
- with sour or acid risings: **NP**

- with 'all gone' feeling: **KP**
- with nervous anticipation: **KP, MP**
- from overindulgence or rich food: **NS**
- with motion: **KP**

Vomiting*:
- after cold food/drinks: **CP**, *MP*
- sour, curdled milk (infant): **CP, NP**
- bile, bitter or green: **NS**
- thick, white or stringy phlegm: **KM**
- undigested food: **FP**
- watery: **NM**

Abdominal symptoms

Abdomen*:
- bloated (gas): **KS**, *MP, NS*
- cramp: **MP**
- cutting pains: **NS**, *NP*
- distended: **MP, NS**
- hardness: **MP**
- tender to touch (pain): **KP**
- swollen: **KM**

Anus*:
- cracks and fissures of: **CF**
- fistula in: **S**, *CF, CS*
- itching (and burning) at: **NP**, *FP*
- pain in: **KM**
- abscess (discharging): **CS**
- prolapse: **CF**, *KP*
- warts: **KM**, *NS*

Colic*: **MP**
- better from warmth: **MP**
- with eating: **CP**
- with much flatulence: **NP, MP**
- with worms: **NP**
- in infants: **MP, CP**

Haemorrhoids*: **CF**, *NS*
- bleeding: **FP**, *CF*
- inflamed and painful: **FP**, *CP*
- itching: **KP**, *CF, NP*
- stinging: **NM**, *CF*
- hernia*: **CF**, *S, CP*

Organ congestion*: **NS, KM**
Organ inflammation or
swelling*: **FP, KM**
Prolapse of rectum*: **CF,** *KP*
Rectum, pain or pain with
• stool*: **MP,** *KM*
• spasm: **MP**

Stool description
Constipation:
• with dull, heavy headache: **KM,** *NM*
• children and aged: **CP**
Creamy*: **NP**
Diarrhoea*:
• after a chill: **FP**
• after fatty food: **KM**
• after vaccination: **KM,** *S*
• alternating with constipation: **NM**
• aggravated by eating fruit: **CP**
• early morning must rush
  from bed: **NS**
• from fright, anxiety, worry etc.: **KP**
• in teething children: **CP**
• with jaundice: **NP**
• with pus or blood: **CS**
Difficult to expel: **S,** *CF*
Dry, crumbly: **NM**
Expelled with force: **MP**
Foetid and foul: **KP**
Green: **NS**
Hard: **NM,** *NS*
Hot: **CP**
Inability to expel*: **CF**
Involuntary*: **KM**
Jelly-like: **NP**
Light or clay coloured*: **KM**
Loose: **NS**
Painful*: **FP**
Receding: **S**
Slimy: **KS**
Undigested: **FP,** *CP*
Watery: **NM**

Whitish*: **KM**
Yellow*: **KS**

Urinary symptoms
Brick dust (red) sediment*: **NS**
Burning after urination:*: **FP,**
NM, NP
Catarrh*: **KM**
Constant urge to urinate (acute)*: **FP**
Cystitis*:
• acute: **FP, KM**
• chronic: **KM**
Enuresis, nocturnal*: **MP,** *KP*
Inflammation*: **FP**
• chronic: **KM,** *CF, FP*
Excessive flow of watery urine*: **NM**
Frequency from nervousness: **KP, MP**
Gravel*: **NS**
• pain in passing: **NS, MP**
• sediment and/or with gouty
  symptoms: **NS, NP**
Incontinence*: **CF**
• weakness of sphincter: **FP**
• paralysis of sphincter: **KP**
Involuntary emission with
exercise*: **NM**
Sandy deposits in urine: **NS**
Spasms or spasmodic retention*: **MP**
Urine, acid*: **NP**

Female symptoms
Aching*: **CP**
Bearing-down pains: **CF,** *FP*
Burning*: **KM, FP**
Congestion*: **KM**
Discharge*:
• albuminous: **CP**
• blackish-red: **KP**
• creamy: **NP**
• greenish: **KS**
• honey-coloured: **NP**
• inflammation (redness): **FP**

- itching and rawness: **NP**, *KM*
- milky-white: **KM**
- thick-white: **KM**
- thick, yellow, bloody: **CS**
- watery, slimy: **NM**
- yellow: **KS**

Menstruation*:
- with back pain: **CP**
- with colic: **MP, CP**, *KP*
- with constipation: **S**, *NS*
- with clotting: **KM** (dark), **FP** (light red)
- with cramping (labour like) : **MP, CP**
- delayed: **KM**
- with diarrhoea: **NS**
- excessive: **KM**, *CF*
- with excitability and nervousness: **KP**
- with extreme coldness: **S**
- with heavy weight in abdomen: **KS**
- retarded or delayed in teenagers: **KM, NM**
- repressed: **NM, KP**
- scalding, acid: **NP**
- sour smelling: **NP**
- thick-white: **KM**
- thin with offensive odour: **KP**
- with weepiness (and sadness): **KP, NM**

Prolapse, uterine*: **CF, CP**
Sterility, glandular causes*: **KM**

Male symptoms

Discharge*:
- albuminous: **CP**
- prostatic fluid: **KM**
- also refer to characteristic discharge of each tissue salt

Inflammation (with swollen prostate)*: **KM, FP**

Induration*: **S, CF**
Scrotum, oedema*: **NS**
Testicles*:
- aching in: **KM**
- indurated: **CF, S**
- swelling: **KM**, *CP*

Weakness after coitus: **KP**

Pregnancy support

Aching in limbs: **CP**
After-pains: **FP, CF**
Cramps: **MP, CP**
Lactation tonic: **CP**, *MP*
Morning sickness: **KM, NP**
Mastitis*:
- first stage (with heat): **FP**
- swelling: **KM, FP**
- suppuration: **CS**, *S*
Nipples*:
- cracked: **CF**, *S*
- sore (and/or inflamed): **CP, IP**
Tonic: **CP, FP, MP**

Respiratory symptoms

Aching in chest*: **CP**
Breathing*:
- constricted: **MP**
- hurried at illness beginning: **FP**
- laboured: **KP**, *MP*
- nervous: **MP**
- oppressed: **FP, MP**
- painful: **FP**
- short: **FP, MP**
Cough*:
- chronic: **CP**
- croupy: **KM, MP**
- dry: **FP**
- hoarseness: **KS**, *FP*
- inflammatory: **FP**
- irritating: **FP**
- nervous: **MP**

- paroxysmal (fits of coughing): **MP, KM, CP**
- painful: **FP**
- with sharp, shooting pains: **MP**
- spasmodic: **MP**
- with teething: **CP**
- tickling: **CP**, *KM*
- worse warm or stuffy room: **KS**

Expectoration*:
- albuminous: **CP**
- blood-streaked: **FP**, *CS*
- clear: **NM**, *KM*
- difficult: **NM, KM, MP**
- greyish-white: **KM**
- greenish: **KS**
- golden-yellow: **NP**
- salty: **NM**
- slimy, sticky and yellowish: **KS**
- small, yellow, and hard lumps: **CF**, *S*
- watery: **NM**
- white: **KM**
- yellow-green, slimy: **KS**

Heat*: **FP**

Pain in chest*: **KM**
- sharp shooting pain: **MP**

Rattling in chest:*: **KM**, *NM*

Spasm*: **MP**

Stiches: **FP**

Sweat at night associated with respiratory ailment*: **CP**

Wheezing*: **KM**

Circulatory symptoms

Anaemia*: **FP**, *CP*

Blood vessels*:
- dilation: **CF**
- constricted: **KM, MP**
- enlarged: **CF**
- inflamed: **FP**
- relaxed: **CF**
- weak: **CF**

Circulation poor*: **CP**, *KP, FP*

Cold extremities: **CP**, *KP, FP*

Fever*: **FP**

Heart*: **KM**, *CF, FP, MP*

Palpitation*:
- with anxiety: **KP, MP**
- from indigestion: **NP**
- with nervousness: **KP, MP**
- with sadness: **KP**

Pulse*:
- felt all over body: **NM**
- full and rapid: **FP**
- irregular: **KP**, *NM, MP*
- weak: **KP**

Varicose*:
- veins: **CF**, *FP*
- ulcerations: **CF**

Structural symptoms, including back

Aching*: **CP**

Coldness: **NM**, *CP*

Bones*:
- bruised: **FP**
- deformed: **S**, *CP, CF*
- deposits: **S**, *CF, NP, NS*
- inflamed: **FP, KM**
- porosity: **CP, MP**, *S*
- soft, fragile: **CP**, *S*
- ulceration: **S**, *CS*

Dislocations*: **CF**

Development slow*: **CP**

Gout*: **NP, NS**

Joints*:
- cracking of: **NP**
- enlarged (indurated) **CF, S**
- hypermobile (relaxed): **CF**
- inflamed **FP, KM**, *CF*
- sprained (Strained): **FP, CF**
- stiffness: **S**, *CF*
- swollen: **KM**, *CF*
- weak: *CF*

Nails brittle or crippled: **S**
Numbness, feeling of*: **CP, KP**
Pain*:
- aching: **CP**
- better by gentle movement: **KP**
- boring or shooting pain: **MP**
- growing pains: **CP**, *MP*
- shifting pains: **KS**
- spasm-related: **MP, CP**
- worse from motion: **S**, *KP*

Paralysis*: **KP**
Sciatica*: **MP, KP**
Shin soreness*: **CP**
Sprains: **FP, CF**
Stiffness (general) **FP**, *KP*
Strains **FP, CF**

Skin including facial symptoms

Abscess*:
- hot, red and painful: **FP**
- pustular: **S**, *CS*

Acne rosacea*: **CP, KM, FP**
Acne, white content: **KM**, *CP*
Atrophy of tissue*: **KP**, *CP*
Bedsores*: **KP**
Blisters*:
- with fetid, watery contents: **KP**
- with clear, watery contents: **NM**

Blotches (red) come and go quickly: **NP**
Boils*: See abscess
Bruises easily: **FP**
Burns*: **KM**
- with blistering: **NM, KM**
- when suppurating: **CS, KM**

Burning sensation of skin: **KS**, *NP*
Chaffed skin: **NS**, *NP, FP*
Cracks in skin: **CF**
Cysts*: **CP**
- indurated: **CF**, *S*
- pustular: **CS**

Dandruff: **KS, NM, KM**
Dryness (general): **CP, NP, KM**
Dryness (patches or areas): **NM**
Elasticity lacking: **CF**
Eruptions*:
- after vaccination: **KM**
- from stress and nervousness: **KP, MP**
- with inflammation: **FP**, *KM*
- with swollen glands: **KM**

Exudations*:
- acid, excoriating: **NP**
- albuminous: **CP**
- clear, thin and watery: **NM**
- golden-yellow: **NP**
- offensive-smelling, fetid: **KP**
- pustular, purulent and often blood-streaked: **CS**
- pustular, thick and yellow: **S**
- white and fibrinous: **KM**
- yellowish and slimy or watery: **KS**

Glands enlarged: **KM**
Greasy skin (general): **KP**
Greasy facial skin (with dry body): **NM**
Hard calloused skin: **CF**, *S*
Healing*:
- pustular tendency: **CS**
- scarring tendency: **S**
- slow: **S**

Herpetic eruptions*: **NM**, *CP*
Hives: **NP**
Inflammation*: **FP, KM**
Ingrowing toenails (or hairs)*: **S**, *KM*
Itching: **CP, NP**, *KM*
Nettle-rash: **NM**, *NP*
Perspiration*:
- lack of: **KS**, *S*
- excessive (especially feet): **S**
- Pimples: **CS, CP**
- all over body: **NP, KM**
- blind: **S**

- barbers' or shaving rash: **CS**
- under beard: **CS**

Rawness of skin: **NP**, *FP*

Scales*: **KM**, *NS*
- from a sticky base: **KS**

Shingles*: **NM**, *KP, MP, FP*

Tinea*: **KS**, *S*

Ulceration*:
- inflamed: **FP**
- not healing: **CF**
- purulent: **CS**
- also refer to 'Exudations'

Vesicular eruptions*:
- with yellowish water: **NS**
- with clear water: **NM**

Warts: **KM**, *CP*

Withered skin*: **KP**

Wrinkles: **CP**
- and sagging: **CF**, *KP*

Eating: **NS**

Eating fatty food: **KM**

Eating fish: **NS**, *NM*

Eating fruit: **CP**

Eating pastry: **KM**

Evening: **KS**, *NP*

Exercise prolonged: **KP**, *FP*

Exertion*: **KP**

Heated atmosphere: **KS**

Full moon: **S**

Motion:*: **KP**

Night: **S**, *CP*

Noise: **KP**, *S*

Rainy weather: **NS**

Rising suddenly from sitting*: **KP**

Seaside (salty atmosphere): **NM**

Thunderstorm: **NP**

Touch: **MP**

Water: **NS**, *CS*

General conditions affecting symptoms

Symptoms aggravated by:

Afternoon: **NP**, *NS*

Change of weather: **CP**, *CF*
- to damp: **NS**

Cold application: **MP**, *CP*

Cold weather: **S**, *NM*

Damp weather or conditions: **NS**, *CP*

Draughts: **MP, CP**

Symptoms relieved by:

Bending double: **MP**

Cold: **FP**

Company (pleasant): **KP**

Cool, open air: **KS**

Eating: **NM**

Excitement: **KP**

Gentle motion: **KP**, *FP*

Heat: **MP**, *CF, S*

Lying down: **CP**

Massage and physical pressure: **MP**

For further information on courses (including by correspondence or email), workshops and private consultations contact:

Mark Wells
P. O. Box 79
Kew East, Vic. 3102
Australia
www.wellsnaturopathy.com.au

NOTES